DIABETES WEIGHTLOSS

Week by Week

JILL WEISENBERGER, MS, RD, CDE

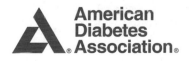
American
Diabetes
Association.

Director, Book Publishing, Abe Ogden; Managing Editor, Greg Guthrie; Acquisitions Editor, Victor Van Beuren; Editor, Courtney Rutledge; Production Manager, Melissa Sprott; Composition, ADA; Cover Design, Drop Cap Design; Illustrations, KTB Studios, LLC; Printer, Victor Graphics.

Printed in the United States of America
1 3 5 7 9 10 8 6 4 2

The suggestions and information contained in this publication are generally consistent with the *Clinical Practice Recommendations* and other policies of the American Diabetes Association, but they do not represent the policy or position of the Association or any of its boards or committees. Reasonable steps have been taken to ensure the accuracy of the information presented. However, the American Diabetes Association cannot ensure the safety or efficacy of any product or service described in this publication. Individuals are advised to consult a physician or other appropriate health care professional before undertaking any diet or exercise program or taking any medication referred to in this publication. Professionals must use and apply their own professional judgment, experience, and training and should not rely solely on the information contained in this publication before prescribing any diet, exercise, or medication. The American Diabetes Association—its officers, directors, employees, volunteers, and members—assumes no responsibility or liability for personal or other injury, loss, or damage that may result from the suggestions or information in this publication.

♾ The paper in this publication meets the requirements of the ANSI Standard Z39.48-1992 (permanence of paper).

ADA titles may be purchased for business or promotional use or for special sales. To purchase more than 50 copies of this book at a discount, or for custom editions of this book with your logo, contact the American Diabetes Association at the address below, at booksales@diabetes.org, or by calling 703-299-2046.

American Diabetes Association
1701 North Beauregard Street
Alexandria, Virginia 22311

DOI: 10.2337/9781580404549

Library of Congress Cataloging-in-Publication Data
Weisenberger, Jill.
  Diabetes weight loss-- week by week : a safe, effective method for losing weight and improving your health / Jill Weisenberger.
     p. cm.
  Includes bibliographical references and index.
  ISBN 978-1-58040-454-9 (pbk.)
  1. Diabetes--Diet therapy. 2. Diabetes--Exercise therapy. 3. Weight loss. 4. Self-care, Health. I. Title.
  RC662.W37 2012
  616.4'620654--dc23
                           2012003694

CONTENTS

ACKNOWLEDGMENTS

Countless people helped me conceive of this book and make it a reality.

First, thanks go to my patients, who have taught me about their lives, struggles with their weight and food choices, and the strategies to their many successes. You all inspire me.

Thank you to all of the wonderful people at the American Diabetes Association, especially to Victor Van Beuren for your relentless support, guidance, and enthusiasm for this project and for always saying something that makes me laugh. To Greg Guthrie, thank you for tirelessly plowing through the details and being such a pleasure to work with.

Many colleagues have contributed to this book. Thank you, Wendy Jo Peterson, MS, RD, Rita Grandgenett, MS, RD, and Judy Doherty for creating such delicious and nutritious recipes. Thank you, Carly Sopko, RD, for helping with recipe testing and making it a fun week together in the kitchen. To Michelle Voss and Sarah Waybright, MS, RD, thank you both for your kind research support, creative minds, and attention to detail. Thanks go to many more colleagues around the country for generously sharing their skills and knowledge and for introducing me to their patients who are profiled in this book.

Nothing in my life would be worth doing without the support of my best friend and husband, Drew Weisenberger. Thank you for always putting me first and for treating me like a princess even though I know I don't deserve it. To Erin and Emily, I thank you both for being terrific daughters and also for putting up with tasting the same recipes over and over and complaining very little. Thank you also for always saying that you are proud of me and for pushing me to do my best the same way I push you to do yours. To my four-legged best friends— Nikki, thanks for making sure I never sat still too long, and Cocoa, thanks for always keeping me company, no matter the time of day or night.

Introduction

GETTING STARTED

Chances are good that you have tried to lose weight in the past—perhaps many times. You may have lost weight but gained it back, plus more. Maybe you stopped losing weight after dropping just a few pounds. Many people with diabetes think it's impossible to control both their weight and blood glucose at the same time and are confused about which one to make a priority. But there's good news; you really can do both. Dealing with the immediate effects of exercise and food choices on your blood glucose does make weight loss more challenging, but it's not impossible.

Why should you be successful this time when you weren't successful in the past? This book does not promote a one-size-fits-all diet. You are not identical to anyone, and your diabetes and your life are not identical to anyone else's either. Therefore, you need to make your own best diet. There are no rules here—just guidance. In *Diabetes Weight Loss—Week by Week*, you'll learn that weight loss is about skill, not willpower. There is a large gap between being motivated and successfully losing weight. That gap needs to be filled with knowledge, strategies, skills, self-confidence, and feedback. That's what this book will give you. By taking small steps, you *can* trim down and feel fabulous—while taking care of your diabetes at the same time. You will learn skills to handle yourself in the kitchen, grocery store, and restaurants. You'll learn to handle tough situations and difficult people. You'll be able to set realistic weight-loss and lifestyle goals, and you'll create ways to be more active.

Having a strong set of skills is far better than having willpower. Think about when you learned to parallel park your car, throw a curveball, or tie your shoes. Did willpower make you successful? Of course not. If you are able to do those things well, it's because you practiced and developed those skills. Becoming a pitcher, bowler, tennis player, cook, or safe driver requires knowledge, strategy, practice, skill, and feedback, either from a coach or your own experiences.

Success also requires that you have the proper attitude. It is important that each week you focus on the knowledge, skills, and strategies that will get you to your weight-loss and health goals. Pay attention to your weight, but don't let that be your focus. Don't be in a rush to lose the weight. By working hard at lifestyle changes, not only will you be healthier and slimmer, you'll also be more likely to keep the weight off and maintain your new healthy habits. That's why this book covers a full year. You'll have plenty of time to practice new skills. You will face new challenges as the seasons change, especially during celebrations, vacations, and other events that occur during a year. This book is designed to reflect the struggles and topics you could work on with a registered dietitian, health coach, or diabetes educator over 12 months. It is advised you see a registered dietitian to help you develop an individualized meal plan based on your personal carbohydrate needs and medications. This book will supplement your plan.

In this week-by-week guide, you will cover a lot of material in the early chapters. There are mini lessons covering diet, food knowledge, cooking skills, behavior change, physical activity, and diabetes-specific concerns. Each chapter covers just a few of these topics. This will give you a good knowledge base that you can translate into actions at a reasonable pace. You must take action, though. Just passively taking in the information is likely to do little to help you change behaviors. Read the sections, practice the skills, decide how you can apply the information. Then, start using your new skills. Each week and month builds on the previous mini lessons. The later chapters provide information and skills for making your weight-management plan work over the long haul.

If you have a burning desire to read ahead to learn more about a particular topic, go ahead. Just as if you were working one-on-one with a registered dietitian, you should cover the topics most important to you. However, you should resist the temptation to take on more than a few topics and skills at one time. Long-term success requires re-learning behaviors, and we can learn only so much at one time. Also, resist the temptation to skip sections. If you are looking to lose weight, everything in this book applies to you.

Share this book and what you learn with your family and others who are important to you. Allow them to support you, and allow them to learn as well. Most of the skills you will learn are the same skills anyone—with diabetes or not—needs to achieve successful weight loss and optimal health. Ask someone who wants to lose weight to work through the book with you. You'll both benefit and enjoy each other's support.

PREPARE TO BE SUCCESSFUL

Before you even get started, ask yourself why you want to lose weight. What is your reason? What motivates you? One benefit of weight loss is better health, which leads to improved control of blood glucose and blood pressure, increased fertility, healthier pregnancies, and reduced risk of heart disease, cancer, and more. Some benefits are directly related to your quality of life: you have more energy, sleep more soundly, cross your legs more comfortably, suffer less knee pain, and wear trendier clothes.

Motivation comes and goes, so you will need to help it along sometimes. Get a jump on that now while your motivation is high. Put together an individualized Motivation Kit. Get a box or notebook or both to collect photos, magazine articles, motivational sayings, meaningful quotations, your list of reasons to lose weight, affirmation cards, and anything else that pumps you up and reminds you of the reasons why you want to get healthier. Keep your Motivation Kit handy so you can reach for it whenever you need it, and so you can add to it often.

WEIGH IN

Use a reliable scale to measure your weight. Plot your weight on the Weight-Loss Graph on page 162 in the Appendix. Do this each time you weigh in. To check the reliability of your scale, weigh yourself three times within a minute or so. Each weight should vary by no more than a pound. If, for example, the scale indicates that you weigh 180 pounds, but when you stand on it two more times it indicates your weight to be 184 and 177 pounds, it's not a reliable scale. Either buy another or plan to regularly visit your doctor's office or gym for your weigh-ins.

How often should you weigh yourself? That depends on you. If you can use the scale as nothing more than information to guide your actions, weigh in at least once a week. This way, you can reevaluate your diet and exercise plan if your weight isn't dropping. But if the number on the scale becomes a source of anxiety rather than merely a number that carries no judgment, weigh yourself less frequently—once a week, once a month, or not at all.

SET SMART GOALS

"I want to lose 15 pounds this week," is an example of an unrealistic goal. *"I plan to lose 1–2 pounds this week,"* is far more realistic but still ineffective. The problem with this statement is that it focuses on the end result and not on the behavior needed to get there. *How* are you going to lose those pounds? What behaviors do you need to change?

"I will eat better," does focus on a behavior—eating. However, it is still too vague to be effective. How do you define eating better? How will you determine if you are successful? Each of these elements needs to be part of your goal.

By following the SMART principles of goal setting, you'll be able to march down a clear path to success. Once you have your goals clearly defined, write them down and keep them in a place where you'll be able to read them often. Below are the five elements of a SMART goal; you will also find a corresponding worksheet in the Appendix on page 165.

S: Specific

Avoid vague goals. Be specific about what you will do, how you will do it, and where you will do it. If your goal is specific, anyone who reads it will know exactly what you plan to do.

M: Measureable

Can you measure your success? Will you be able to report if you are 100% or 75% successful?

A: Action Oriented

Be certain your goal is listed as a behavior. What action will *you* take?

R: Realistic

Is this goal attainable if you put forth effort? Can you achieve this with the resources you have?

T: Timely

Know when you will do this and when you will assess your results.

EXAMPLES OF SMART GOAL SETTING

Vague	SMART
I will eat better	This week, I will eat 1 cup of fruit and at least 2 cups of vegetables every day. **AND/OR** I will not skip any meals this week.
I will eat less.	At dinner, I will serve myself my usual portion of food, but only once, no second or third helpings.
I will exercise more.	I will walk for at least 30 minutes at least five times this week or exercise for a total of at least 150 minutes. If the weather is bad, I'll use the treadmill or an exercise DVD.

Once your goals are written, ask yourself what you need to do to be successful. If you plan to eat fruits and vegetables with every meal, you'll need to have them on hand. If you regularly skip breakfast, you might need to set your alarm to get up 20 minutes earlier each day or prepare a grab-and-go breakfast the night before. By thinking through your goals clearly, you're setting yourself up to win.

Now you're ready to begin. Be prepared to work hard, plan ahead, and learn new skills.

Part 1

THE BASICS IN 16 WEEKS

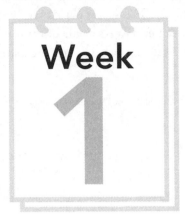

Week 1

Week 1 addresses the most basic skills you need in order to start losing weight that you can keep off forever. You will learn that calories rule, about the importance of keeping records, that there is more than one way to eat healthfully, and how to get active.

CALORIES RULE

With so much talk about fats and carbohydrate in the media and among friends, the simple calorie gets neglected. In fact, many people don't fully understand what a calorie is, and many people ignore them completely. Technically, a calorie is a unit of energy. We need calories from food to run our bodies, just like a car requires energy from gas in order to operate. If we take in more energy than we need, it gets stored as fat and we gain weight. The only way to lose weight is to consume fewer calories than the body uses. Fats and carbs are important, but they are not what matters most when it comes to your weight.

The amount of calories your body needs depends on many things: your weight, the amount of muscle and fat you have, your activity level, genetics, and more. This number is neither good nor bad; it's just a number. Think of it the same way you consider the yards of fabric you need to cover your windows or the number of bricks you need to build a house. Different types and sizes require different amounts.

You don't have to count calories to drop pounds, but it's important to know your approximate calorie needs so you can decide how particular foods and their portions fit into your eating plan. Visit ChooseMyPlate.gov, a site created by the U.S. Department of Agriculture (USDA), where you'll enter your age, weight, and activity level to learn how many calories you need to lose weight. Generally, women require 1,200–1,800 calories per day for weight loss, and men need about 1,600–2,400 calories per day. As a rule of thumb, most women should not consume fewer than 1,200 calories per day, and men should stay at 1,600 calories or more.

||||||||||||||||||||||||||||||||||||||||||||||||||||||||||||||||||||||||||||||||||||||||||||||||||||||||||||||||||||||||||||||||||||||||||||||||||||||||||||||||||

TIP!

To lose one pound of fat, you must cut back or burn an extra 3,500 calories.

||||||||||||||||||||||||||||||||||||||||||||||||||||||||||||||||||||||||||||||||||||||||||||||||||||||||||||||||||||||||||||||||||||||||||||||||||||||||||||||||||

Make a few simple changes daily to start whittling away calories. Below are a few ideas for trimming your plate, and you'll find more specific suggestions during Week 5. Incorporating these simple changes into your daily routine will help you get to your goal.

+ Pare down your meat and starch servings 10–20% by leaving several bites on your plate or by serving yourself just a little less.
+ Cook with a little less oil. Use a little less salad dressing or use a low-calorie salad dressing.
+ Spread more mustard than mayonnaise.
+ Trade in a large bagel for a medium-sized English muffin.
+ Switch from whole milk to low-fat or nonfat milk.
+ Eat reduced-fat cheese, yogurt, and sour cream in place of the regular versions.
+ Drink coffee and tea without sugar.
+ Drink water or other zero-calorie beverages instead of soda, punch, or fruit juice.
+ Remove chicken skin.
+ Trim the fat from red meats.
+ Bake, broil, or grill instead of frying.

To learn more about the calories in your foods, refer to food labels, pick up a pocket-sized calorie counter at the bookstore, and visit websites like *ChooseMyPlate.gov* and *MyFoodAdvisor.com*.

Although calories directly affect weight, monitoring fats and carbs is also important to your health. As a general rule, you should be able to consume at least 45 grams of carbohydrate at each meal with no more than a 40-mg/dl rise in blood glucose from your first bite at a meal until two hours later. If you need additional diabetes medications, or if you do not currently take any medications and find that you're having trouble with your blood glucose, talk with your doctor or nurse. You need balanced meals to lose weight healthfully, enjoy your food, and prevent the complications of diabetes and other health problems, so keep tabs on your blood glucose and adjust your carbohydrate intake as needed.

EXAMPLE

Sample Meal Containing about 45 Grams of Carbohydrate

2 slices whole-wheat bread (30 grams) with sliced chicken, reduced-fat cheese, roasted red peppers, lettuce, tomato, onion, and mustard
1 medium peach (15 grams)
Unsweetened iced tea, artificial sweetener if desired

Blood glucose before eating: 103 mg/dl
Blood glucose two hours after the first bite: 138 mg/dl
138 mg/dl – 103 mg/dl = 35 mg/dl
This is acceptable because the change in blood glucose is less than 40 mg/dl.

BE AWARE. BE VERY AWARE

Food records work. Writing down your food intake can double your weight-loss success, according to research funded by the National Institutes of Health. In a study of nearly 17,000 people, those who recorded their daily calorie intake lost twice as much weight as those who kept no records. The simple act of recording your food choices increases your awareness and makes you accountable to yourself. Grab a notebook or buy a journal and get started. Look at the example on the next page to see how it's done. There's a blank food record on page 167 in the Appendix.

Time/Meal (Place)	Food, Amount, Preparation	Blood Glucose, Physical Activity, & Other Notes
7 am/Breakfast (Home)	6 ounces black coffee Quick oats, prepared with water, 3/4 cup cooked 1 tsp honey 2 Tbsp raisins 1 hard-boiled egg with salt	Fasting blood glucose: 119, just a little hungry
10 am/Snack (Office)	Diet yogurt, 6 ounces	Regular break time
11:30 am (Office)	2 mini candy bars	Not planned and not hungry, everyone else at work was eating them
1 pm/Lunch (Break room)	2 ounces turkey on 2 slices whole wheat with mustard Lettuce, tomato, bell pepper on sandwich 12 ounces unsweetened iced tea	Regretting chocolate attack
3 pm	------------------------	Blood glucose: 173
5:30 pm (Car, driving home)	2 granola bars	Very hungry
6:45 pm/Dinner (home)	1 slice meatloaf 3/4 cup mashed potatoes (no gravy) 1 cup green beans	
7:30 pm	------------------------	20 minute walk
9:15 pm	1/4 cup ice cream	Couldn't resist when others were eating, had just a little.
11:20 pm/Bedtime	------------------------	Blood glucose: 141

Record your intake as you go through the day, even if you have to use scratch paper and rewrite it or tape it into your journal later. Don't wait until the end of the day to jot everything down. It's easy to forget what you've eaten or to fall a few days behind. Waiting may also mean that it's easier to give in to temptation. Having to reach for your journal and a pencil will make you mindful of the five French fries you could grab from your spouse's plate and all of the other mindless nibbles that add up to quite a lot over time. Each day, review your food record and try to learn from it. Look for patterns of overeating or mindless munching. Then, take steps to do better tomorrow.

BILL K'S STORY

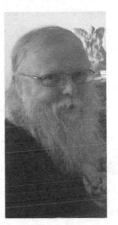

" I keep a very detailed Excel spreadsheet that captures time of meal, blood glucose, medications, carbohydrates, calories, and more. I know this sounds like a bit too much documentation for many who are struggling with diabetes, but the more information you can share with your medical team, the better they can help you. And by documenting my carb and calorie intake, I can determine how much I can eat at each meal so I don't exceed my prescribed intake. "

HIGH CARB OR LOW CARB?

A lot of people ask, "How many carbs should I have each day or how much fat should I eat to lose weight? What diet is best?"

The truth is that there's probably no best diet. Some people have very strong opinions, but there are good arguments for many diet plans. Some people lose weight and manage their blood glucose on very-high-carbohydrate vegetarian diets. Others eat meat with most meals and prefer less carbohydrate. Some people use the glycemic index or another ranking method to help them select food. The plan you choose must be one that works with your life and your preferences, but it must also include a variety of wholesome foods from the various food groups, with special attention to including whole grains and a variety of colorful fruits and vegetables. Additionally, you'll need to tweak your diet periodically based on your blood glucose levels, cholesterol, blood pressure, and other health markers.

The USDA and U.S. Department of Health and Human Services jointly publish their *Dietary Guidelines for Americans* every five years and provide helpful nutrition information and recommendations for all Americans. The 2010 edition includes four healthful meal patterns (which are described in the Appendix), including USDA meal patterns, vegetarian and vegan adaptations, and the DASH (Dietary Approaches to Stop Hypertension) eating plan. A fifth meal pattern, the Mediterranean eating style, is also featured in the *Dietary Guidelines for Americans*. You can learn more about the Mediterranean diet at Oldways (www.oldwayspt.org) and in *The Mediterranean Diabetes Cookbook* by Amy Riolo (American Diabetes Association, 2010). In short, the Mediterranean diet includes fruits, vegetables, and whole grains at most meals. Beans and fish are important sources of protein, and nuts, seeds, olives, and olive oil provide good-for-you fats. Cheese and yogurt are eaten regularly, but in small amounts, and herbs and spices—not salt—season foods. If you haven't done so yet, now is a great time to see a registered dietitian (RD) for an individualized diet plan. Visit eatright.org to find an RD in your area.

TIP!

If you choose to use the glycemic index to help plan your meals, keep in mind that it's best to use it in conjunction with another meal-planning method, such as carb counting. You can learn more about the glycemic index at www.glycemicindex.com or by reading *The Low GI Shopper's Guide to GI Values 2011: The Authoritative Source of Glycemic Index Values for 1200 Foods,* by Dr. Jennie Brand-Miller and Kaye Foster-Powell.

START MOVING

If you're not already active, it's time to start. Assuming you're relatively healthy, you can begin walking. If you're unsure, have complications of diabetes, or want to begin something more vigorous than walking, get the go ahead from your health care team first.

Physical activity is perhaps the best medicine available. It makes weight loss easier by burning extra calories. It also improves blood glucose control and cholesterol levels, lowers blood pressure, reduces the risk for heart disease and other chronic diseases, relieves stress, and improves quality of life. Guidelines issued jointly by the American Diabetes Association and the American College of Sports Medicine call for individuals with type 2 diabetes to engage in brisk walking, or other moderate to vigorous aerobic exercise, at least three times per week for a total of 150 minutes or more and to engage in strength training exercises two to three times a week. Don't jump right in. If you're not used to strenuous activity, start off slowly. For example, take several 5-minute walks over the day.

What Is Exercise?

A complete exercise program consists of each of the following components.

Aerobic: activities that use large muscle groups and cause you to breathe heavily as you take in more oxygen; improves fitness of the heart and lungs; good for burning calories

✦ Walking, swimming, jogging, biking, skating, dancing, cross-country skiing

Strength: activities that use repeated movements against resistance; builds and tones muscle; increases strength

✦ Weight lifting, resistance bands, pushups, lunges, sit ups

Flexibility: increases ability of a joint to move through a full range of motion

✦ Stretching, yoga, Pilates

Balance: strength, flexibility, and other activities that improve coordination and help you prevent falls

✦ Standing on one foot, sitting on an exercise ball, yoga

The table below shows the approximate number of calories burned by individuals with different weights. Get moving!

Physical Activity	Calories per Hour 140-lb person	Calories per Hour 190-lb person
Walking 3.0 mph (20-minute mile)	210	285
Walking 4.0 mph (15-minute mile)	318	432
Jogging 5.2 mph (11.5-minute mile)	572	778
Running 7.5 mph (8-minute mile)	795	1,080
Bicycling 12–13.9 mph	509	691
Aerobic dancing, low impact	318	432
Aerobic dancing, high impact	445	605
Weight lifting/power lifting	382	518
Water aerobics/calisthenics	254	346
Bowling	191	259
Ballroom dancing, waltz, foxtrot	191	259

Source: *The Compendium for Physical Activities Tracking Guide* (2000)

Using a Pedometer

Walking is a favorite exercise among people who want to lose weight. Increase your motivation by using a pedometer. A pedometer is a handy little device that you carry in your purse or pocket or clip to your pants that counts each and every step you take while you are wearing it.

+ Expect to spend about $30.00 for a reliable pedometer. Some are very fancy and have lots of additional functions, but the only must-have feature is its ability to count steps.

+ Start off with the pedometer clipped to your waistband above the center of your knee. To check its accuracy and to find the best placement, set your pedometer to zero. Wiggle and bend a little. A good pedometer will measure steps only, not twists and turns. Next, with your pedometer still set at zero, walk exactly 100 steps. If your pedometer registers between 90 and 110 steps, consider it accurate. If it appears to be inaccurate, move it to other places on your waistband and continue checking until you find the right spot. If your pants roll down at the waistband or are very loose, try turning the pedometer inward so it faces your body. If moving the pedometer to various places doesn't make it count your steps accurately, you should return it and select a different brand.

+ Wear your pedometer all day for several days to determine your average number of steps. Then set a goal to increase your average number of steps by 500 to 2,000 steps daily. A typical long-term goal is 10,000 steps per day.

Exercising with Diabetic Eye Disease or Nerve Disease

Though the benefits of being active are almost always greater than the risks, some complications of diabetes may restrict your choice of activities. If you have proliferative retinopathy (eye disease), then exercises that increase blood pressure (such as high-intensity aerobics and weight lifting and activities that jar the head or place the head below the level of the heart) may damage your eyes further. Check with an ophthalmologist for advice before beginning any exercise routine.

Peripheral neuropathy (nerve disease) can cause numbness, pain, and weakness in the hands and feet. Though physical activity can help prevent or ease neuropathy, if you have a foot injury or ulcer, talk to your doctor about appropriate exercises and avoid weight-bearing activities, such as walking and dancing. Stick to swimming and biking and take extra care to protect your feet. If you have autonomic neuropathy, which affects the heart, lungs, stomach, intestines, bladder, or genitals, you must obtain physician approval and receive specific guidance before exercising.

||||||||||||||||||||||||||||||||||||||||||||||||||||||||||||||||||||||||||||||||||||||||||||||||||||||||||||||||||||||||||

TIP!

Whenever you exercise, especially if you are alone, wear a medical ID bracelet or carry identification that states you have diabetes and lists your medications and an emergency contact. If you can, carry a cell phone and blood glucose meter as well.

||||||||||||||||||||||||||||||||||||||||||||||||||||||||||||||||||||||||||||||||||||||||||||||||||||||||||||||||||||||||||

MEDICATION CHECK

Some diabetes medications, as well as other medications such as prednisone, certain antidepressants, and beta-blockers, may make weight loss difficult. If you're taking one of these or another you think may cause weight gain, ask your health care provider to review your drugs. Perhaps you can take an alternate medication or lower your dose. No matter what, don't make changes without discussing it first with a member of your health care team.

WEEK 1 ACTION STEPS

Select from the following goals or steps, modify them, or create your own. Choose the ones that are important to you while being careful not to overwhelm yourself with more than you can handle. This week I will:

☐ Make 2 SMART goals.

☐ Record my food intake and activity daily.

☐ Learn my calorie needs at *www.ChooseMyPlate.gov*. My calorie needs are _____.

☐ Use a calorie-counting book/website to estimate my intake.

☐ Decrease my calorie intake in the following ways:_____

_____

☐ Learn more about the Mediterranean diet by visiting *www.oldwayspt.org*.

☐ Speak to my health care provider about beginning an exercise program.

☐ Increase my weekly physical activity by 45 minutes.

☐ Determine my baseline daily steps by wearing a pedometer.

☐ Other: _____

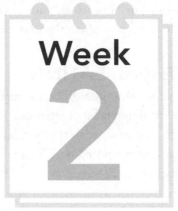

Week 2

Now that you know some basics about calories and several balanced meal plans, you'll learn a few guidelines for planning your meals, how food labels can help you stay on track, and how your blood glucose might change with your new diet. But first, you'll pick a weight-loss goal.

PICK A WEIGHT-LOSS GOAL

To get healthier you don't need to lose tons of weight. Dropping as little as 5–10% of your starting weight is a big plus. Losing just a little can significantly lower your LDL (bad) cholesterol, reduce your risk for certain cancers, lower blood pressure, and may help you control your blood glucose with fewer medications or lower doses. If needed, start with a goal to lose 10% of your starting

Your Weight (pounds)	10%(pounds)	New Goal Weight (pounds)
140	14	126
160	16	144
180	18	162
200	20	180
220	22	198
240	24	216
260	26	234
280	28	252
300	30	270
320	32	288
340	34	306
360	36	324

weight (see the table on the previous page). Once you hit that mark, in say, 3–6 months, decide if you want to work toward an additional 5–10%. Beginning with a small goal, such as losing 5 pounds in the first month, is a good idea.

WHAT IS HEALTHFUL EATING?

Eating healthfully shouldn't be complicated. It's not easy in our fast-paced, fast food society, but a healthful nutrition prescription shouldn't be difficult to understand or be filled with lists of strict or tricky rules. Unfortunately most diet plans found on the Internet and promoted on TV are complicated, unbalanced, or both. Many have long lists of foods to eat and longer lists of foods that you shouldn't eat. Some require that you avoid carbohydrates or eat them only at certain hours. Others forbid fats. Some require combining one food group with another. All of this is more complicated than necessary, and it doesn't usually lead to good nutrition or lasting weight loss. Often individuals who follow a plan like this eventually return to old eating habits and regain all of the lost weight plus more!

Refer to any of the five meal patterns discussed in Week 1 and the Appendix for descriptions of healthful eating, or simply get started with these guidelines for uncomplicated nutritious eating.

✦ Spread your food out over the day. Eat at least three meals daily.
✦ Include the foods you love, but be smart about how often you eat them and about portion sizes.
✦ Eat more foods derived from plants than from animals—this means more fruits, vegetables, nuts, whole grains, and beans than meats and cheese.
✦ Choose foods as close to their natural state as possible. Limit highly processed foods.
✦ Aim for three or more food groups per meal.
✦ Eat a variety of food groups and a variety within each food group.
✦ Limit added sugars, solid fats, animal fats, and excess sodium.

By following these guidelines, you'll know what to put in your grocery cart and what to prepare for dinner. You'll come home from the supermarket with wholesome fruits, vegetables, whole grains, lean meats, and low-fat dairy. Most of these foods will look as nature provided them rather than like they came from a food processing plant. You don't have to avoid them completely, but you'll limit foods like cookies, candy, chips, stick margarine, boxed macaroni and cheese, seasoned rice mixes, instant soups, sodas, processed meats, and more. Take inspiration from the 7 day menus in the Appendix on page 183. Don't feel that you need to follow these menus exactly. They couldn't possibly meet the preferences and schedules of all readers. Rather, they are here as one more tool to offer you guidance and motivation.

TIP!

When planning your meals and snacks, include foods that will keep you from getting hungry again quickly. Most people find satisfaction when they combine protein-rich foods like low-fat Greek yogurt, tofu, eggs, and poultry with fiber-rich foods such as vegetables, whole grains, and fruits.

PLATE METHOD

Perhaps the simplest meal planning strategy at home is the Plate Method, which guides both your choices and your portions. Start with a 9-inch plate. Draw an imaginary line down the middle, and fill half the plate with non-starchy vegetables like broccoli, tomatoes, carrots, zucchini, and green beans. Divide the other half between a small portion of lean meat, such as chicken, fish, or beef, and a small portion of a starchy food, such as pasta, rice, bread, or starchy vegetables like peas. Add a cup of low-fat milk and a small piece of fruit for dessert and your meal is complete.

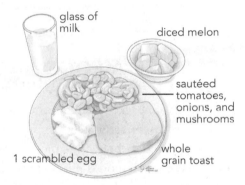

glass of milk

diced melon

sautéed tomatoes, onions, and mushrooms

1 scrambled egg

whole grain toast

You can use the same principles for breakfast, though you might omit the vegetables. You could also keep the vegetables by having a breakfast pizza or by topping your egg and toast with jarred salsa. See the Appendix (page 168) for a Weekly Plate Method Planner.

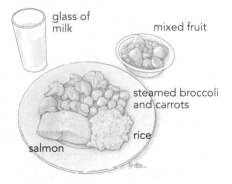

glass of milk

mixed fruit

steamed broccoli and carrots

rice

salmon

FOR MORE INFORMATION ABOUT HEALTHFUL EATING:

ChooseMyPlate.gov: *www.choosemyplate.gov*

Create Your Plate: American Diabetes Association: *www.diabetes.org/ food-and-fitness/food/planning-meals/create-your-plate/*

Dietary Guidelines for Americans: *www.cnpp.usda.gov/dietaryguidelines.htm*

Your Guide to Lowering Your Blood Pressure with DASH
(Dietary Approaches to Stop Hypertension): National Heart Lung and Blood Institute: *http://www.nhlbi.nih.gov/health/public/heart/hbp/dash*

The Vegetarian Resource Group: *http://www.vrg.org*

Vegetarian Nutrition Dietetic Practice Group of the Academy of Nutrition and Dietetics: *http://www.vegetariannutrition.net*

|||||||||||||||||||||||||||||||||||||||||||||||||||||||||||||||||||||||||||||||||||||||||||||||||||||||||||||||||||||||||||||||||||||||||||||

DECIPHER A FOOD LABEL: PORTION VS. SERVING SIZE

Food labels are packed with information to help you control your weight and blood glucose. Unfortunately, many people underestimate the calories, saturated fat, sodium, and carbohydrate they eat, even when they look at food labels. The reason? Too much food is piled on the plate. Portion sizes and serving sizes are not the same thing. A portion of food is the amount we eat. A serving is the amount listed on the food label. If your portion is two or three servings, you need to double or triple the calories, carbs, and everything else to estimate the amount you will actually eat. There's too much error in guessing. Even people who are certain they can't be fooled find that they also underestimate the amount they eat.

Serving sizes in restaurants, single-serve packages, and even cookbooks have ballooned in recent decades, so most of us have some degree of portion distortion. To get a good handle on the amount of calories you eat, you need to use food labels, a calorie-counting book or website, measuring cups, and a food scale. As an experiment, pour out your usual amount of cereal or scoop out your usual portion of pasta. Then measure it and compare it to the serving size. Do this with all types of foods: chips, fruit, meats, everything. The results will probably surprise you.

Serving Size: Everything on the label is for this amount of food, so look here first.

Calories: If you ate the full can of soup, your calorie intake is 125 × 2, or 250 calories. (Calories affect your weight. Consider how this fits into your total daily calorie allotment.)

Servings Per Container: Definitely check this out. It's easy to mistake the package size for the serving size. This is especially tricky with small packages like canned soups, bags of chips, and bottled drinks.

Carbohydrate: Eating the full can doubles your carbohydrate intake to 48 grams. (Carbohydrates affect your blood glucose after eating. Consider how this fits into your meal allowance.)

VEGETABLE AND PASTA SOUP

Nutrition Facts

Serving Size 1 cup (240 mL)
Servings Per Container About 2

Amount Per Serving

Calories 125   **Calories from Fat** 10

	% Daily Value**
Total Fat 1g	2%
Saturated Fat 0g	0%
Trans Fat 0g	
Cholesterol Less than 5mg	2%
Sodium 480mg	20%
Total Carbohydrate 24g	8%
Dietary Fiber 6g	24%
Sugars 0g	
Protein 6g	

*Percent Daily Values are based on a 2,000 calorie diet. Your Daily Values may be higher or lower depending on your calorie needs.

		Calories:	2,000	2,500
Total Fat	Less than		65g	80g
Sat Fat	Less than		20g	25g
Cholesterol	Less than		300mg	300mg
Sodium	Less than		2,400mg	2,400mg
Potassium			3,500mg	3,500mg
Total Carbohydrate			300g	375g
Dietary Fiber			25g	30g

Calories per gram:
Fat 9   •   Carbohydrate 4   •   Protein 4

MONITOR BLOOD GLUCOSE OFTEN

Now that you're eating better, and possibly beginning to lose weight, your body might be handling carbohydrate better than it did before. This is a good thing, but it may put you at greater risk of having low blood glucose (hypoglycemia), especially if you take certain diabetes medications. Hypoglycemia is when your blood glucose level is less than 70 mg/dl. You may or may not experience symptoms, so don't fall into the trap of thinking you don't need to check. Not all diabetes medications can cause hypoglycemia. Insulin and some of the diabetes pills can. To see how your new diet affects you, test your blood glucose more often than usual. A list of times to self-monitor your blood glucose (SMBG) is given below. Choose the times and the frequency that give you the information you need. If you usually check twice daily, you may want to start checking at least four times now and whenever you make big changes in diet or exercise. Share your SMBG results with your health care team and ask if your diabetes medications should be changed as you lose weight.

+ Before meals and two hours after the start of the meals
+ Bedtime
+ 3 a.m.
+ Before and after exercise
+ Whenever you feel shaky, dizzy, nervous, lightheaded, confused, or dis-oriented (symptoms of hypoglycemia)

WEEK 2 ACTION STEPS

Continue your current goals or rewrite them if necessary. Additionally, select from the following goals or steps, modify them, or create your own. Choose goals from the previous week if applicable. This week I will:

☐ Continue the following goals: _____ _____

_____ _____ _____

_____ _____ _____

☐ Aim to lose 1–2 pounds.

☐ Record my food intake and activity every day.

☐ Use the Plate Method for meals.

☐ Use a dinner plate no larger than 9 inches.

☐ Use measuring cups whenever I eat cereal, rice, pasta, potatoes, and other starches.

☐ Use measuring cups whenever I eat the following types of food:

_____ _____ _____.

☐ Read labels for every food I eat.

☐ Eat at least two fruits and three vegetables every day.

☐ Use food labels and other tools to help me with my calories and portions.

☐ Decrease my calorie intake in the following ways:_____ _____.

☐ Check my blood glucose at least _____ times each day.

☐ Not skip any meals.

☐ Take a 10-minute walk at least twice a day.

☐ Add 1,000 steps to my daily step goal.

☐ Other: _____ _____ _____

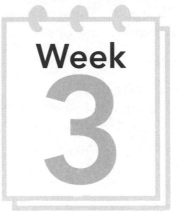

Week 3

All that healthful eating we've been talking about starts with a good breakfast, so this week you'll learn why it's so important and how to put one together in no time. We'll cover more tips to trim calories, build on your walking program, and make use of your food record.

EAT BREAKFAST

Rush! Hurry! Go! There's no time for breakfast!

Hey, not so fast! A little planning will help you get a balanced morning meal lickety-split. You may wonder why you should eat breakfast when you're trying to lose weight. It's simple; skipping meals causes people to overeat. Eating breakfast is a critical strategy for weight loss and the prevention of weight regain, though many who skip breakfast have the misguided notion that it saves them calories. Many of those who are certain that they are not eating more calories overall when they skip breakfast really are. Among participants in the National Weight Control Registry (NWCR)—a listing of thousands of people who have lost at least 30 pounds and kept if off for at least one year—78% eat breakfast every day. Additionally, eating breakfast is associated with healthier cholesterol levels, better insulin sensitivity, and greater intakes of several vitamins and minerals, including potassium, calcium, iron, and vitamin C.

If you're worried that eating in the morning will raise your blood glucose, you'll be delighted to see how eating may actually push those morning numbers down. Morning blood glucose levels are largely regulated by hormonal factors and the actions of your liver. While sleeping, your cells use up the glucose from your dinner or evening snack, so the liver sends more glucose into the blood.

Often in type 2 diabetes, the liver doesn't recognize that there is ample blood glucose available, so it sends more out. Eating a food with carbohydrate tells the liver that you are no longer fasting, so it stops releasing extra glucose.

BREAKFAST IN A SCRAMBLE

✦ Start your day with a piece of fruit, if the thought of eating in the morning makes you queasy. Eventually add other food groups.

✦ Get organized the night before.
- Pack a peanut butter and banana sandwich and a cup of low-fat milk to go.
- Measure out dry cereal and store it in the refrigerator with a cup of low-calorie yogurt and a plastic spoon to take with you.
- Prepare your own trail mix of dry whole-grain cereals, dried apricots, dried cherries, and other favorite dried fruits. Pair with a cup of yogurt, or if you want to avoid more carbohydrate, grab a tiny container of cottage cheese, or a cheese stick to round out this speedy breakfast.

✦ Keep a few meal-replacement bars and drinks on hand for when all else fails. Keep some at home and at work.
- Pick those with at least 3 grams of fiber, 10 grams of protein, no more than 3 grams of saturated fat, and about 250–400 calories. See Week 13 for more information about meal replacements.

✦ Make a smoothie with nonfat Greek yogurt and frozen fruit. Eat it at home or take it with you. See the recipe for Mixed Berry Smoothie in the Appendix (page 200).

✦ Stock up on dry and cooked whole-grain cereals. If you prefer long-cooking oats, prepare several servings at once. Store the leftovers in the refrigerator in serving-size containers.

✦ Early in the week, make several hard-boiled eggs. In the morning, grab one, along with toast or fruit or both.

✦ Scramble eggs with diced peppers and onions. Wrap them in a tortilla or place between two halves of an English muffin.

✦ Combine any three food groups such as grains, lean meat, and fruit, if you don't like traditional breakfast foods,

✦ Eat last night's leftovers.

CHERYL S'S STORY

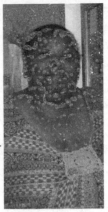

" I always thought I was too busy to eat breakfast, and I thought that skipping breakfast would mean less calories overall. But, that wasn't true. Eating breakfast has helped me control my blood glucose better and has kept me from getting so hungry that I eat whatever is convenient. What's really surprising is that I feel SO much better. Now I plan ahead to get my breakfast ready while I'm getting ready for work. I even keep some things in the freezer for days when I'm in a hurry. Eating regularly throughout the day is one of the best things I can do for myself. "

USE A SMALL DISH

Eating behavior expert Brian Wansink, Ph.D., author of *Mindless Eating: Why We Eat More Than We Think We Eat* (Bantam Dell, 2006), argues that on average Americans eat about 30–35% more than they think they do. Even the most aware individuals eat about 20% more than they realize. If you think you aren't influenced by the size of a dish, you probably are, he says. When nutrition science professors and graduate students were given various sizes of ice cream scoops and bowls to serve themselves at a party, those with the larger dish served up to 127 more calories compared with those with the smaller dish. That amount increased further when they had both the larger dish and the larger scoop. Even students and professors who know lots about food and what they are eating can be misled!

If the size of a dish can trick you into eating more, it can also trick you into eating less. Apply this concept to all aspects of eating and drinking. Will it be more satisfying to eat a 4-ounce steak on a 12-inch dinner plate or on an 8-inch salad plate? On the bigger plate, the steak looks like a child's serving. Pull out your small dishes and glasses or buy some attractive new ones. Use nothing larger than a 9-inch plate for dinner, 1-cup bowls for cereal, ½-cup dishes for ice cream and other desserts, and 1-ounce shot glasses for M & M's, jellybeans, and the like.

KEEP MOVING

For weight loss, blood glucose control, and overall fitness, you should engage in both cardiovascular (aerobic) and strength-training exercises. If you have any doubts about beginning an exercise program, or about cranking it up a notch if you're already active, talk to your physician first. If you started walking last week or just started wearing a pedometer, keep it up this week and do a bit more, if possible. Our emphasis this week is on cardiovascular exercise. Walking, swimming, biking, stair climbing, dancing, and other activities that get you breathing heavily for several minutes strengthen your heart. This type of activity aids weight loss by burning calories, giving you a boost in energy (this is why being tired is a poor excuse not to exercise), improving triglyceride and cholesterol levels, increasing insulin sensitivity, and lowering blood glucose levels.

You may feel overwhelmed with the recommendation to engage in at least 150 minutes of cardiovascular activity weekly. If so, take it slowly. Any amount of activity is better than none. Thirty minutes is better than 20, and 20 minutes is better than 10. Set SMART goals for exercise, just as you do for dietary changes. Examine where you are, where you want to go, and make strategies to get there. The best activity to pick is the one you enjoy, and the best time to do it is the time that works for you. For example, if exercising before bed makes it hard to relax into a good slumber, you might be more consistent if you exercise before dinner. Be sure to pick an indoor activity for bad weather days as well.

During exercise, you should work hard enough to improve fitness, but not so hard to hurt yourself. Warm up for a few minutes with some slow walking and some gentle stretches before beginning your aerobic activity. Do something similar after your activity. Adjust your intensity up or down to hit the range you are aiming for. As your fitness improves, add either a few minutes to your exercise routine or pick up the intensity a bit. Listen to your body and follow the pace that's right for you.

Rate Your Exercise

A useful tool to help you judge your exercise is the Borg Rate of Perceived Exertion (RPE) Scale. It helps you assess your level of effort. The Borg Scale ranges from 6 to 20. Generally, a rating between 12 and 14 indicates a moderate level of intensity.

Here's how you use it: while doing physical activity, rate how you perceive your level of exertion. Consider how strenuous the exercise feels to you, including your sense of exertion, effort, and fatigue. Focus on your whole body's level of exertion, not just on any one part of your body. Then, choose the number on the scale that best represents how you perceive your level of effort.

The Borg Scale runs from 6 (no exertion at all) to 20 (maximal exertion). A 9 is "very light" exertion, such as an easy, slow walk. At 13, the effort is "somewhat hard," the work is tiring but you can keep going on. For 15, you're working out pretty hard, and at 17, the physical activity is strenuous and tiring. When you get up to 19, it's hard to consider keeping up this level of exertion for any length of time.

It's important to try to honestly assess your exertion level. Don't think about how difficult you think the activity should be. Just scan your body and fairly assess how hard it is working. Honest assessments will yield the best results. For more information, check out this website: *www.cdc.gov/physicalactivity/everyone/measuring/exertion.html.*

AVOID LOW BLOOD GLUCOSE DURING AND AFTER EXERCISE

Both losing weight and becoming more active improve insulin action. If you use insulin or any of the pills that sometimes cause low blood glucose, exercising puts you at risk for hypoglycemia both during the activity and for as long as a full day later. To avoid exercise-induced hypoglycemia, follow these guidelines.

+ Measure your blood glucose before starting to exercise. If it's below 100 mg/dl AND if you take medications that can cause low blood glucose, you will need a snack of about 15 grams of carbohydrate or whatever amount is necessary to raise your blood glucose to 100 mg/dl. A small piece of fruit will usually do. If you take no diabetes medications, it is unlikely that you need a snack.

+ If you are exercising at a very high intensity, doing interval training, or doing intense weight training, you may need a carbohydrate-containing snack both during and after exercise to help prevent hypoglycemia some hours later.

✦ Measure your blood glucose frequently before, during, and after exercise to learn how different activities uniquely affect you. Check whenever you feel like your blood glucose is low.

✦ Always carry a source of carbohydrate in case you experience hypoglycemia. Follow the Rule of 15 if your blood glucose ever drops below 70 mg/dl.

- If you have your blood glucose meter, use it. If your blood glucose is less than 70 mg/dl, or if you don't have your meter but believe your blood glucose is low, consume 15 grams of carbohydrate. It's best to use pure glucose in the form of tablets, gel, or liquid because it works quickly and contains a minimum of calories. Some good choices include:
  - 2–5 glucose tablets (check the label for the proper dosage)
  - 1 tube of glucose gel
  - 2 tablespoons of raisins
  - 4 ounces of regular soda or fruit juice
  - 1 tablespoon of sugar or honey
  - 1 cup of nonfat or low-fat milk

  Do not use candy bars and desserts because they add calories, saturated fats, and work slowly. If that is all you have, however, use it.

- The second half of the Rule of 15 is to wait 15 minutes after treating before eating anything else or resuming activity. Measure your blood glucose again. If it's still low, consume another 15 grams of carbohydrate.

- Recheck your blood glucose in another 15 minutes. Continue to treat with 15 grams of carbohydrate and recheck in 15 minutes until your blood glucose is back to normal.

- If your next meal is hours away, you may need a snack.

MORE FROM BILL K

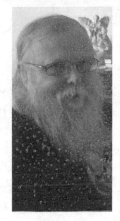

" Exercise is a big part of my diabetes management and weight-loss plan. Sometimes when I'd exercise, though, my blood glucose would go too low, which forced me to take in extra carbs to push it back into my target range. Weight loss is difficult under any circumstances, but being forced to eat to keep my blood glucose up was making it a lot harder. I worked with a certified diabetes educator, who is also a registered dietitian, to help adjust my insulin dose, so my blood glucose wouldn't go too low. That did the trick. By reducing my insulin, I was able to eat less, which reduced my calorie intake. Weight loss is definitely achievable with persistence. "

REFLECT ON YOUR FOOD RECORD

You've kept your food record for at least two weeks by now. Take some time to look at it carefully. What patterns do you see? Perhaps you've noticed that you eat mindlessly in front of the television or feel the need for sweets in the afternoon. Maybe you tend to take second and third helpings, even though you've had enough to eat. Do you eat too fast, without fully tasting your food? By monitoring your own behaviors and progress, you can identify problem areas and take note of the strategies that work for you and those that do not. Some people like to review their food record daily and to write notes about things they did well or not so well. Then, they set a goal for the next day. Other people prefer to reflect on their food records weekly. Do what you prefer and what works for you and put those SMART goal practices into action.

FRANK P'S STORY

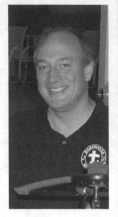

66 I keep a food record with a computer program that calculates my intake of calories, fat, protein, and carbohydrates. This helps me see if I'm on track or falling away from my goals, and it helps me feel like I have some control. For example, if I see that I'm going to go over my calorie budget for the day, I can choose what to do. I can choose to eat different foods or eat less or hit the gym a bit harder to balance things out.

I've had a few AHA! moments. Sometimes I feel as if I haven't eaten very much during the day, but then I see that the calories, fats, or carbohydrates were significantly higher than I thought they were. Usually in those situations, I realized I gave myself excuses for eating something earlier and only fooled myself. Keeping records helps me see what I'm really doing and guides me to make good choices. 99

WEEK 3 ACTION STEPS

Continue your current goals or rewrite them if necessary. Additionally, select from the following goals or steps, modify them, or create your own. Choose goals from the previous weeks if applicable. This week I will:

☐ Continue the following goals: _____

_____

_____

☐ Record and reflect on my food intake daily.

☐ Not skip any meals.

☐ Keep the following foods on hand to make eating breakfast easier:

_____

_____.

☐ Use a smaller plate for dinner and small dishes at other times.

☐ Add 1,000 steps to my daily step goal.

☐ Wake up 20 minutes earlier to fit in a few minutes of physical activity.

☐ Pull out my old exercise DVDs.

☐ Check my blood glucose before, during, and after exercise.

☐ Carry a source of glucose with me when I exercise.

☐ Other:_____.

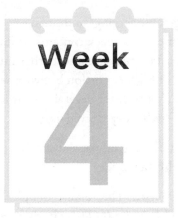

Week 4

This week you will expand on your meal-planning skills and put more emphasis on including foods that keep hunger at bay. You'll also build on the food label lesson from Week 2, when you examined the serving sizes. In this chapter, you'll learn to evaluate some of the claims made on labels and to compare two similar products. Finally, you'll make a plan to reward yourself.

EAT WATER-RICH FOODS

Eating more can actually help you lose weight!

Any diet plan that leaves you hungry will be short lived. Success comes when you find an eating plan that consists of tasty foods that both trim overall calories and fill the belly. Fortunately, there's no shortage of delicious and filling low-calorie foods. Those are the foods you need to go after. What makes a food filling? One thing that keeps hunger away is eating water-rich foods, like vegetables, fruits, and soups. The water that's naturally present in fruits and vegetables adds volume to food, giving you a bigger, more satisfying portion than if the water was not present. Consider this example: which is more filling, 15 grapes or 15 raisins? The grapes come out on top due to their high water content.

Generally, vegetables are a better calorie and carbohydrate bargain than fruits, so focus more on veggies. Starting your meal with a low-calorie salad is a smart strategy. It helped women in a study at Pennsylvania State University eat fewer calories than when they ate a high-calorie salad or no salad at all before their entrée. Broth-based soups also work quite well. Avoid creamy soups, though, because the fat in the milk or cream adds calories to the soup.

Your options are endless. For example:

- ✦ Double your vegetable servings at dinner.
- ✦ Make sure each meal and snack contains fruits, vegetables, or both.
- ✦ Add veggies to pastas, casseroles, and other mixed dishes so you can have your usual (or bigger) portion but with fewer calories.
- ✦ In the winter, warm up with a vegetable or minestrone soup. In the summer, cool off with a cup of cold gazpacho.

You'll learn more about bulking up your meals to trim calories in Week 10. The following books are also helpful.

- ✦ *The Ultimate Volumetrics Diet: Smart, Simple, Science-Based Strategies for Losing Weight and Keeping It Off*, by Barbara Rolls, PhD, with Mindy Hermann, RD
- ✦ *The Volumetrics Weight Control Plan: Feel Full on Fewer Calories*, by Barbara Rolls, PhD, and Robert A. Barnett
- ✦ *The Volumetrics Eating Plan: Techniques and Recipes for Feeling Full on Fewer Calories*, by Barbara Rolls, PhD

400-CALORIE LUNCHES

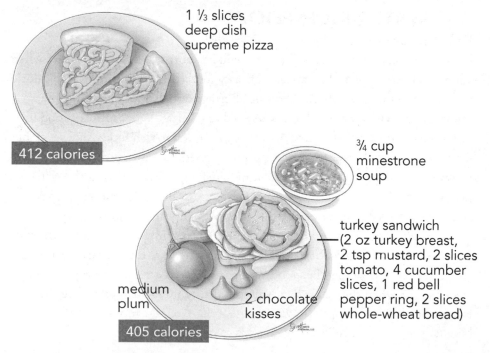

1 ⅓ slices deep dish supreme pizza

412 calories

¾ cup minestrone soup

turkey sandwich (2 oz turkey breast, 2 tsp mustard, 2 slices tomato, 4 cucumber slices, 1 red bell pepper ring, 2 slices whole-wheat bread)

medium plum

2 chocolate kisses

405 calories

FAT-FREE ISN'T FREE

Evaluating foods based on the front of the package is a common trap for shoppers trying to eat well. Big letters with words like "Free," "Less," "Reduced," and "Low" lure us in. They sound good, but are they? Sometimes yes, and sometimes no. Here are some things to consider:

- ✦ Does the food provide good nutrition or is it simply lower-fat junk food?
- ✦ How do the calories and carbohydrates fit into your meal plan?
- ✦ How do the sodium, saturated fat, and other components of the food fit into your meal plan?
- ✦ Does the modified food taste good?
- ✦ How does the cost compare to the regular product?

The key to avoiding this common trap is to examine the Nutrition Facts panel. It takes a little bit longer than just glancing at the front of the packaging, but it is a necessary step. Consider the food labels below. When you compare 1% low-fat milk with whole milk, you can see that the 1% milk is a much better bargain in calories and saturated fat. Making the switch from whole milk to 1% milk saves you 40 calories and 3.5 grams saturated fat in each cup. The cholesterol content is significantly lower in the low-fat milk as well. The amounts of sodium, carbohydrate, and protein are similar in the two products, making the low-fat milk a much better choice.

WHOLE MILK		
Nutrition Facts		
Serving Size 1 cup (240mL)		
Servings Per Container About 8		
Amount Per Serving		
Calories 150	Calories from Fat 70	
		% Daily Value*
Total Fat 8g		12%
Saturated Fat 5g		25%
Cholesterol 35mg		12%
Sodium 125mg		5%
Total Carbohydrate 12g		4%
Dietary Fiber 0g		0%
Sugars 12g		
Protein 8g		
Calories per gram:		
Fat 9 • Carbohydrate 4 • Protein 4		

1% MILK		
Nutrition Facts		
Serving Size 1 cup (240mL)		
Servings Per Container About 8		
Amount Per Serving		
Calories 110	Calories from Fat 20	
		% Daily Value*
Total Fat 2.5g		4%
Saturated Fat 1.5g		8%
Cholesterol 13mg		4%
Sodium 125mg		5%
Total Carbohydrate 13g		4%
Dietary Fiber 0g		0%
Sugars 12g		
Protein 8g		
Calories per gram:		
Fat 9 • Carbohydrate 4 • Protein 4		

Now look at the two labels for fig bars below. The difference between these two is far from impressive. The calorie difference is just 10 calories, and there is little difference in anything else. In fact, the sodium and carbohydrate levels are slightly higher in the fat-free bar. What's more, neither product offers much in the way of nutrition. You might think the bar is nutritious simply because it contains figs. Yes, figs are nutritious, but there must not be much fig in these bars since the fiber content is so low. Fig bars are cookies, and fat-free fig bars are fat-free cookies. Now that's not to say that you shouldn't eat them. If you really like them, work them into your meal plan. Just recognize that they're not a health food and be certain to account for the carbohydrates and calories in whichever variety you choose, just like you do with any other food.

FIG BAR

Nutrition Facts

Serving Size 1 bar
Servings Per Container 2

Amount Per Serving

Calories 110	**Calories from Fat** 20
	% Daily Value*
Total Fat 2g	3%
Saturated Fat 0g	0%
Cholesterol 0mg	0%
Sodium 135mg	6%
Total Carbohydrate 22g	7%
Dietary Fiber 1g	4%
Sugars 12g	
Protein 1g	

Calories per gram:
Fat 9 • Carbohydrate 4 • Protein 4

FAT-FREE FIG BAR

Nutrition Facts

Serving Size 1 bar
Servings Per Container 2

Amount Per Serving

Calories 100	**Calories from Fat** 0
	% Daily Value*
Total Fat 0g	0%
Saturated Fat 0g	0%
Cholesterol 0mg	0%
Sodium 145mg	6%
Total Carbohydrate 23g	8%
Dietary Fiber 1g	4%
Sugars 12g	
Protein 1g	

Calories per gram:
Fat 9 • Carbohydrate 4 • Protein 4

REWARD YOURSELF

Congratulations! You're approaching one month since you started eating more healthfully and exercising with purpose. You deserve a reward. Whether we're celebrating a promotion, an unexpected windfall, a child's acceptance to college, or a few lost pounds, it's tempting to reward ourselves with dessert, dinner out, or an extra glass of wine. Food rewards not only feed us with extra calories, they also perpetuate the notion that indulgent food is nurturing. It's time to come up with a list of nonfood rewards. Here are a few ideas to get you started.

- ✦ Listen to music.
- ✦ Buy a new song for your mp3 player.
- ✦ Spend a few minutes outside reading or simply watching the birds.
- ✦ Hire someone to clean your house, mow your lawn, or do any other chore you'd be thrilled not to do.
- ✦ Treat yourself to a spa day—either at home or at a real spa.
- ✦ Schedule an extra date night or night out with friends.

WEEK 4 ACTION STEPS

Continue your current goals or rewrite them if necessary. Additionally, select from the following goals or steps, modify them, or create your own. Choose goals from the previous weeks if applicable. This week I will:

☐ Continue the following goals: _____

_____

_____

☐ Record and reflect on my food intake daily.

☐ Double my vegetables at each dinner.

☐ Start at least one meal daily with a broth-based soup or low-calorie salad.

☐ Learn new healthy ways to cook vegetables.

☐ Eat at least two pieces of fruit and have three servings of vegetables daily.

☐ Continue to read food labels for serving size, calories, and more.

☐ Reward myself without food. Instead I will _____.

☐ Add 1,000 steps to my daily step goal.

☐ Review my Motivation Kit and add to it.

☐ Other:_____.

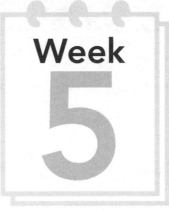

Week 5

This chapter adds to the calorie-trimming tips and strategies that you've learned in previous weeks. You will also learn about adding strength training to your fitness plan and techniques to help you evaluate whether the goals you have chosen are suitable.

FOOD SWAPS

By now, you've practiced reading food labels for calories, carbohydrates, fats, and other things and you've found a few ways to cut back. Some strategies you might not have already considered are shown in the table below.

Instead of This	Do This	Approximate Calories Saved	Bonus
Fruit juice	Eat the whole fruit. One small orange or apple has 60 calories, but 1 cup of juice has about 110.	50	More filling, more fiber, takes longer to eat
Fruit-on-the-bottom yogurt	Add ½ cup fresh fruit to plain low-fat Greek yogurt	40 per 6-oz serving	More filling, less added sugar, higher protein, higher fiber
Broccoli cheese or cream soups	Sip vegetable soup	80 per cup	More fiber, less saturated fat, probably more vegetables
Applesauce, regular	Opt for applesauce without added sugar	50–60 per ½ cup	Less added sugars and carbohydrate
2% milk	Drink skim milk	40 per cup	Less saturated fat

Instead of This	Do This	Approximate Calories Saved	Bonus
Butter	Spread whipped butter or "spreadable" butter (butter and vegetable oil)	30–50 per Tbsp	Less saturated fat, easier to spread when cold
Cream	Whiten your coffee with fat-free half and half	20 per Tbsp	Less saturated fat
Sour cream	Substitute Greek yogurt when making dips	200–220 per 6-ounce container	Higher protein, less fat
Cheese	Omit the cheese on your usual sandwich	100–110	Less saturated fat
	Or		
	Use 1 Tbsp avocado in place of 1 ounce of cheese	50	More fiber and heart-healthy fats
	Or		
	Use 1 oz hummus in place of 1 ounce of cheese	50	More fiber, less saturated fat
Chicken with skin	Remove chicken skin after cooking	Fried: 100 per thigh, 175 per breast / Roasted: 40 per thigh, 50 per breast	Less saturated fat
Prime rib	Enjoy top sirloin steak	65 per 5 ounces	Less saturated fat
Large tortilla	Wrap up with a taco-sized tortilla instead of the burrito-sized one	60–75	Less carbohydrate
Bagel, breads, buns	Downsize them. Choose a small bagel or an English muffin over a large bagel	75–200	Less carbohydrate
Instant flavored oatmeal	Instant unflavored oatmeal	60 per pack	Less sodium and no added sugars
Croutons	Top your salad with fresh herbs and toasted walnuts	60–70 per 1 ounce croutons replaced with 1 Tbsp chopped nuts	More healthy fats, more antioxidants, more flavor

Instead of This	Do This	Approximate Calories Saved	Bonus
Wine	Sip a wine spritzer with equal parts wine and club soda	70 calories per 6-ounce beverage	Less alcohol (alcohol can reduce inhibitions and cause you to eat more than you would otherwise)
Alfredo sauce	Toss pasta or chicken with marinara sauce	120–140 per ½ cup	More vitamins and antioxidants, less saturated fat, more vegetables
Chips	Dip veggies into hummus or salsa	90 per 1-ounce portion of chips replaced with 1 cup of veggies	More fiber and overall nutrient intake, lower fat intake
Regular candy bar	Scale back your candy bar from a regular to a fun size	100–200	Less saturated fat, less added sugars and carbohydrate
Regular soda	Choose water, sparkling/seltzer water, or flavored water over soda	140 per 12-ounce can	Less added sugars and carbohydrate, fewer additives and colors
Apple pie	Enjoy a warm baked apple with cinnamon instead of a slice of apple pie	200 per ⅛ of 9" pie replaced with a baked apple	Less added sugars and saturated fat, more fiber, more antioxidants
Regular mayonnaise	Spread reduced-fat mayonnaise or mustard on your sandwich	55 calories per 1 Tbsp for reduced-fat mayo; 85 calories with mustard	Less fat, more flavor
Pepperoni pizza	Remove the pepperoni from your pizza	10 per piece of pepperoni	Less saturated fat and sodium
Potato chips	Snack on baked potato chips	30 per ounce	Less fat
Finishing your dinner	Leave a few bites on your plate	20–200	Varies
Filling up on starches	Trim your starch servings (rice, pasta, potatoes) by ¼–½ cup	50–120	Less carbohydrate

TO CHANGE OR NOT TO CHANGE?

Knowing what to do isn't the same as knowing how to do it or even wanting to do it. You may feel that it's important to exercise or eat five servings of vegetables each day, but you just haven't made those changes or some other desired changes yet. Sometimes when people aren't successful, it's simply because they chose the wrong goal. Is the goal too large? Does a family member or a doctor tell you it's important, but you don't think it is? There are a lot of reasons your goal might not be the right one for you today. You need to assess both your motivation to work toward your goal and your confidence in being able to achieve it. You are most likely to be successful if you have a moderate to high degree of both motivation and confidence.

Think about your SMART goal. Now look at the diagram below. What number represents your motivation to work on this goal? What number represents your confidence that you can achieve this SMART goal? If you don't rank your confidence as 7 or more, then success may be difficult and you should probably revise your goal. If your motivation is high but your confidence is low, ask yourself why you chose this goal, whether you can achieve this goal at a lower level, what benefit you will gain by reaching this goal, and how important it is. The conversation you have with yourself may guide you to success.

MOTIVATION AND CONFIDENCE RULER

| 0 | 1 | 2 | 3 | 4 | 5 | 6 | 7 | 8 | 9 | 10 |

NOT AT ALL MOTIVATED
OR CONFIDENT

EXTREMELY MOTIVATED
OR CONFIDENT

BUILD MUSCLE

In week 1, you learned about the four components of physical fitness (aerobic, strength, flexibility, and balance), and you were encouraged to start some walking or other aerobic activity. This week, take some time to do at least a little strength-building exercise. Though you'll sometimes hear people say that you should focus on aerobic activity to burn calories, strength training isn't any less essential. Not only does building muscle increase your metabolic rate some (not a lot, but some), it also improves insulin resistance and helps you stay strong for your everyday activities. This becomes even more important as we age and naturally lose muscle mass. Remember, however, that if you have proliferative retinopathy (eye disease), you should not lift weights without the approval of an ophthalmologist.

You don't have to join a gym to get started. Simple push-ups and sit-ups count. So does working with elastic stretch bands, which are available at sports and discount stores. You may, however, find that you enjoy your workouts and get more out of them if you go to a gym or work with a personal trainer to learn proper techniques. In their joint paper, the American Diabetes Association and the American College of Sports Medicine recommend performing 5–10 exercises that involve the upper body, lower body, and core for two to three sessions every week. Start out slowly and work up to this goal.

||||||||||||||||||||||||||||||||||||||||||||||||||||||||||||||||||||||||||||||||||||||||||||||||||||||||||||||||||||||||||||||||||||||||||||||||||||||

LEARN MORE ABOUT STRENGTH TRAINING

■ American College of Sports Medicine (*www.acsm.org*): you can download free exercise brochures.

■ U.C. Berkeley Wellness Letter.com (*www.berkeleywellness.com/html/fw/fwFit03StrengthTraining.html*): description of a basic strength-training session.

■ American Council on Exercise (*www.acefitness.org*): provides an exercise library for various types of equipment or for exercise without equipment.

■ See more about finding and working with a personal trainer in Week 13.

||||||||||||||||||||||||||||||||||||||||||||||||||||||||||||||||||||||||||||||||||||||||||||||||||||||||||||||||||||||||||||||||||||||||||||||||||||||

PANTRY RAID

Set yourself up to be successful! That means not relying on willpower, but instead making plans and using skills. Willpower rarely lasts long, but skills and strategies are yours forever. Try a few of these tricks to create a perfect environment for winning at weight loss.

✦ Instead of keeping tempting foods in sight, "hide" them in hard-to-reach places like the back corner of the pantry or the high cabinet above the refrigerator. At the very least, store them in dark containers.

✦ Buy your family the treats that are easy for you to resist.

- Divide crackers, nuts, cereal, and other foods into healthy portions and put them in individual baggies or containers. Store the baggies in the original box.
- Make it a house rule to keep all junk food away from the home. Anyone who wants a treat can go to the store, ice cream shop, or bakery to buy a single serving.
- If there are foods in your refrigerator or pantry that you want to avoid, store them all on the same shelf. Let others in the house know what belongs there.
- Make snacking on fruits and veggies as easy as grabbing a bag of chips. Place washed cherries, grapes, carrots, cauliflower, and more at eye level in the refrigerator. Keep them in baggies to make them an easy grab-and-go snack.
- If you find yourself snacking all day, prepare limited and appropriate snacks first thing in the morning. At snack time, that's all you have to choose from.

BARBARA C'S STORY

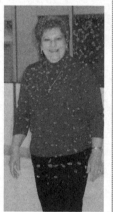

❝ I love ice cream, pies, and cakes, but I don't keep them in the house anymore. If I don't see it, I don't have a hankering for it. I might eat some chocolates or something else when I visit my daughter, and sometimes when I go out, but that's it. It's easier to resist when it's not staring me in the face. ❞

WEEK 5 ACTION STEPS

Continue your current goals or rewrite them if necessary. Additionally, select from the following goals or steps, modify them, or create your own. Choose goals from the previous weeks if applicable. This week I will:

☐ Continue the following goals: _____

_____

_____

☐ Record and reflect on my food intake daily.

☐ Eat vegetables at every lunch and dinner.

☐ Continue to eat breakfast daily.

☐ Use the motivation and confidence diagram with my SMART goals.

☐ Make the following food swaps: _____.

☐ Eliminate all sweet drinks.

☐ Select small, whole-grain bagels and rolls and potatoes at the supermarket.

☐ Replace my regular dairy products with reduced-fat or nonfat versions.

☐ Add at least 10 minutes of strength training to my exercise routine three times a week.

☐ Buy my family the types of sweets and chips that don't tempt me.

☐ Pre-wash fruit and vegetables, and make them readily available.

☐ Add 1,000 steps to my daily step goal.

☐ Other: _____

Week 6

So far, we have covered quite a bit about food choices and exercise, and you have probably made great strides in both areas. Though we touch on physical activity again, this week we discuss two new topics that are important for continued success: the way you may talk to yourself when you've strayed from your diet and weight-friendly techniques for preparing foods at home.

MAKE EXCUSES TO EXERCISE

Do any of these sound familiar? *Too busy. Too tired. Too hot. Too cold. Too windy.* Instead of finding excuses not to exercise (and we all have them), start looking for excuses *to* exercise. What are the tangible benefits that *you* experience when you are physically active? There are health benefits, such as lower blood pressure and improved cholesterol, and there are benefits to the way you feel. Blow off a bad mood with a yoga class or look forward to a sounder sleep with a bike ride earlier in the day. Now is a good time to consider this. Make a written list and put it in your Motivation Kit.

Physical activity is more than structured exercise. Try to increase your activity through both planned exercise and regular daily activities. Think about your day and all of the things that need to get done. Maybe the tasks that could get you moving you instead delegate to others. What chore can you tackle while getting some physical activity? Vacuuming the family room burns more calories than sitting in the family room watching television. Even letting the dogs in and out adds enough steps over several months to make a difference. Instead of asking someone else to tend to the barking, feel good about doing it yourself. This is a different way to look at your day. Practice it enough, and being active will become second nature. Here are some other options for adding physical activity to your day.

- ✦ Beat stress with a 10-minute walk instead of watching TV or reading a magazine.
- ✦ Walk next door instead of picking up the phone. Walk to your coworker's desk instead of calling or emailing.
- ✦ Walk or bike with a friend instead of meeting for lunch.
- ✦ Pace around the house while on the phone or while waiting for a pot of water to boil.
- ✦ Mop or vacuum.
- ✦ Wash and vacuum the car.
- ✦ Play with the kids.
- ✦ Play active video games.
- ✦ Do sit-ups, push-ups, or knee-bends or jump rope during commercial breaks.

RUFUS G'S STORY

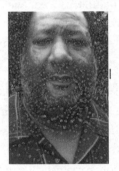

" As an electrician on a university campus, I have to provide services to all of the buildings. I used to ride in a truck instead of walking. Now when I don't need the truck for a large load of materials, I walk all over the campus to get in more steps and burn more calories. I even walk up and down some of the handicap ramps when entering or leaving the buildings to get as many steps as I can. The university has a fitness center too, so I use their treadmill and weight equipment at least three times a week. With all of this exercise and a better diet, my glucose is in the normal range and I lost 60 pounds! "

HALT NEGATIVE SELF-TALK

If you stray from your diet plan or slack off on some goals, you can either beat yourself up or pick yourself up. Which will lead you to your goal? A lot of people are pretty darn hard on themselves after a dietary indiscretion or a few days without exercise. Beating yourself up doesn't help. Really and truly, it doesn't!

Perhaps disappointment or a tiny bit of guilt is beneficial if it spurs you on to do better, but a lot of guilt simply holds us back.

Stop to think about how you talk to yourself when you've strayed from your diet plan. The following scenario is all too common.

||||||||||||||||||||||||||||||||||||||||||||||||||||||||||||||||||||||||||||||||||||||||||||||||||||||||||||||||||||||||||||||||||||||||||||||||||||||||||

Behavior: I ate two slices of birthday cake at work when I planned to have just two bites.

Self-Talk: I can't believe I messed up again. I'm such a pig!! And everyone at work knows it. I'll never lose weight.

Reaction: I've already ruined my diet, so I might as well have stuffed-crust pepperoni pizza for dinner.

||||||||||||||||||||||||||||||||||||||||||||||||||||||||||||||||||||||||||||||||||||||||||||||||||||||||||||||||||||||||||||||||||||||||||||||||||||||||||

In this scenario, the feelings of self-loathing and self-doubt led the dieter further astray. It became a self-fulfilling prophecy. Speaking negatively and making the problem seem unfixable and bigger than it really is kept this person from taking positive action. Let's reverse this trend and see how positive self-talk can be beneficial when you hit a roadblock.

||||||||||||||||||||||||||||||||||||||||||||||||||||||||||||||||||||||||||||||||||||||||||||||||||||||||||||||||||||||||||||||||||||||||||||||||||||||||||

Behavior: I ate two slices of birthday cake at work when I planned to have just two bites.

Self-Talk: I wish I hadn't eaten that. It's not good for my weight, blood glucose, or cholesterol. Plus, I always feel better when I stick to my plan.

Reaction: I'll take a longer walk this evening. Next time, I'll serve myself a tiny piece of dessert and move to the other side of the room before eating.

||||||||||||||||||||||||||||||||||||||||||||||||||||||||||||||||||||||||||||||||||||||||||||||||||||||||||||||||||||||||||||||||||||||||||||||||||||||||||

It's easy to see that the second pattern of thinking is far more productive. It's hard work, however, to change a pattern of thinking that you've been following for most of your life. But once you are there, you will see how liberating it is to be rid of the negativity. So, how can you change your way of thinking? The first step is to pay attention to the words you say to yourself. Once you notice the negative self-talk, step back and observe the situation objectively—like you would if you were watching someone else. Would you be as harsh? Does eating two pieces of cake really mean failure? To help you put it into perspective, ask yourself if this will really matter in three months. If you treat it as the simple mistake it is and move on, then the answer is no, it will not make a difference in three months or even three days. Once you see the situation objectively, the next step is to make a plan to handle a similar situation better next time. Be realistic, though. We all falter, and there will be a next time. Slipping up on your diet doesn't mean you are a failure any more than having a fender bender means you are a dangerous driver.

HOP: CHANGING SELF-FULFILLING PROPHECIES
1. Hear the negative self-talk.
2. Observe the situation objectively as if you were observing a friend.
3. Plan a different response for the next similar situation.

For some people, shifting away from negative self-talk is too difficult to do without help. If you are unable to make progress on your own, seek the help of a mental health professional for support and guidance.

MORE FROM FRANK P.

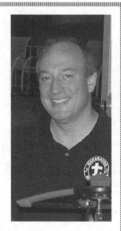

" Food slip-ups are not a big deal in the grand scheme of things. Slip-ups happen often, and realizing it's not a big deal helps me move past it. To keep the slip-up from becoming a total diet fiasco, I think about my two alternatives: a) continue back into old habits that were clearly a problem for me or b) try harder and get back to the basic strategies that bring me success. The solution for me is to muster up self-initiative and motivation by thinking of all the work I've done to get where I am and asking myself if I really want to throw it all away. This is where I reset and use my initial strategies for success to get back on track and to move forward. After all, I've already figured out how to do it and can use that as my tool to find my way back. "

COOK IT!

When you cook your meals at home, you have so much flexibility in what you eat and how it's prepared. At home, you can easily measure your food to estimate the carbohydrates and calories. You can control the sodium and limit the saturated fats. You can pile on the vegetables and eat the combinations of foods you most enjoy.

Traditional recipes tend to load up on calories by using more fat than necessary. Be at least a little stingy with all fat because it's highly caloric. Also, limit trans fats and saturated fats for the sake of your heart (more about that in Month 6). Find ways to use less or choose a different cooking method. For example, deep frying uses more oil than roasting or sautéing. Often a recipe will call for browning meat in several tablespoons of oil, when really just one table-spoon will do. Try these healthy cooking strategies.

✦ Flavor food with fancy vinegars and fresh or dried herbs instead of extra fat and salt.

✦ Cook with nonstick pans.

✦ Spray small amounts of oil into the pan or directly on the food.

✦ Use small amounts of broth, flavored vinegar, or even water to deglaze your pan (scrape up bits of meat or vegetables stuck to the bottom of the pan) instead of using extra oil.

✦ Add complexity to your recipe by browning meats before baking or stewing.

✦ Use smart cooking techniques: baking, braising, poaching, roasting, sautéing, steaming, and stir-frying.

WEIGHT-CONSCIOUS INGREDIENT SUBSTITUTIONS

Instead of This	Try This	Notes
Bottled salad dressing	Reduced-fat bottled salad dressing, or before shaking your bottle, open the lid and pour a small amount of oil out.	
Butter or cheese on a potato or vegetable	Salsa	Great way to get more vegetables, too
Butter, shortening, or oil in baking	Applesauce or mashed prunes for up to half the fat	Baked goods stay moist
Cheddar cheese, 1 cup	¾ cup sharp cheddar cheese	The sharp cheese has a stronger flavor, so you can use less

Instead of This	Try This	Notes
Cream in soups and sauces	Fat-free half and half	Alternatively, thicken soups with a vegetable purée
Mayonnaise	Reduced-fat mayonnaise	Try different brands to find one you like
Nuts, $\frac{1}{2}$ cup	$\frac{1}{3}$ cup toasted nuts	Toasted nuts have a stronger flavor, so you can use less
Oil in marinades	Decrease oil by $\frac{1}{4}$ to $\frac{1}{2}$	Flavored vinegars, citrus juices, and wines also make good marinades
Oil in pan cooking	Sauté in half the oil or use broth. Use cooking sprays and nonstick pans	Zap vegetables in the microwave before sautéing to initiate cooking, finish in pan for added texture and flavor
Poultry with the skin	Poultry without the skin	To keep the meat moist, either remove the skin before eating or use seasoned crumbs on skinless chicken before cooking
Prime rib	Eye of the round	Generally, any cut of beef with "loin" or "round" is a lean cut
Regular ground beef	Ground meat that is at least 90% lean	Read labels for ground turkey. Some are high in calories and fat because it is ground with the skin on
		You can also extend your ground beef by adding lentils, beans, shredded zucchini, or other vegetables
Soups and stews	Prepare soups and stews a day early	Fat rises to the top and hardens, making it easy to skim the fat
Sour cream	Reduced-fat or fat-free sour cream	Avoid fat-free sour cream in savory recipes because it may sweeten your dish
Sugar in baking	Reduce the sugar by $\frac{1}{4}$–$\frac{1}{3}$ or cut sugar in half and use a combination of sugar and sugar substitute	Sweetness can be intensified with the addition of cinnamon, nutmeg, or vanilla extract or by sprinkling a small amount on top just before or after baking

5 Cool Tools for the Smart Cook

Use these to pump up flavor, whittle away at extra fat and salt, and boost nutrition.

1. Gravy separator: Use the flavorful liquid at the bottom of the cup to make your gravy. The high-calorie, high-saturated-fat portion rises to the top. If you do not have a gravy separator, you can do it yourself. Allow the gravy to cool. The fat will rise, allowing you to skim off the fatty portion of the gravy.
2. Zester: Grate citrus zest over plain brown rice or green vegetables. Grate just a smidgeon of Parmesan cheese over your salad or dark chocolate over fresh fruit.
3. Herb scissors: Make easy work of snipping herbs, which are natural flavor boosters.
4. Oil pump mister: Spray your favorite oil into the pan or right onto your food.
5. Immersion blender: Purée small amounts of vegetables, such as potatoes and cauliflower, to thicken sauces and other dishes. Purée carrots, winter squash, or tomatoes right in the cooking pot to make thick, velvety soups without the cream. Use this technique when you prepare Curry Roasted Cauliflower Soup (available in the Appendix on page 201).

BECOME KITCHEN COMPETENT

If you have limited cooking skills, think about giving yourself a SMART goal to learn some practical cooking techniques. Check out local colleges, community centers, and cooking schools to see what's available in your area, or use any of the following books and websites to teach yourself.

- *How to Cook Everything*, by Mark Bittman (book and iPhone app)
- *Cooking Light Way to Cook: The Complete Visual Guide to Everyday Cooking*, by the editors of *Cooking Light Magazine*
- *Cook's Illustrated Magazine* and website (www.cooksillustrated.com)
- Rouxbe™ Cooking School: http://rouxbe.com/myrouxbe

WEEK 6 ACTION STEPS

Continue your current goals or rewrite them if necessary. Additionally, select from the following goals or steps, modify them, or create your own. Choose goals from the previous weeks if applicable. This week I will:

☐ Continue the following goals: _____

_____

_____

☐ Record and reflect on my food intake daily.

☐ Eat vegetables at every lunch and dinner.

☐ Make a list of the benefits from exercise.

☐ Add to my Motivation Kit.

☐ Stop using the phone to speak to colleagues or neighbors when I can walk.

☐ Exercise during at least one set of commercials per day.

☐ Use HOP strategies to stop negative self-talk.

☐ Find and prepare at least three new, healthful recipes.

☐ Remove poultry skin.

☐ Add 1,000 steps to my daily step goal.

☐ Other: _____

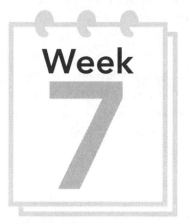

Week 7

We're taking a break from heavy emphasis on food, diet, and activity this week. Rather, as we did in Week 5 in Pantry Raid, we'll look at how switching up your environment can help you break a bad habit, such as over-snacking at night, or start a good habit, such as grabbing fruit instead of chips. Finally, you'll look at additional ways to monitor your changes in behavior and food choices.

TAME NIGHTTIME NIBBLES

Both weight and blood glucose are difficult to control for people who eat a lot of their calories in the evening. For those who rarely eat a full meal during the day, the evening is often filled with extra-large portions and too many calories, carbohydrates, and fats. Then, with so much food at night, breakfast the next morning isn't even on the radar, and the cycle continues. Rein in nighttime overindulgences with these strategies.

✦ Start spreading your calories evenly throughout the day. If you really can't stomach breakfast, have a piece of toast, a handful of dry cereal, or a cup of light yogurt a couple hours after waking. Eat a moderate-sized lunch and a light afternoon snack. End your evening with a moderate-sized dinner and one planned snack. Keep working on this until you are hungry for breakfast and not over-hungry in the evenings. Be patient; it can take a few weeks.

✦ Change your nighttime routine. If you're used to snacking in front of the TV in the den, move upstairs to watch in another room. Even moving to another part of the room might help you break the TV-snack habit. Even better is to spend your evening doing something other than watching television. If you're going to snack, limit its size and focus on enjoying it.

✦ Close the kitchen once you've had your dinner or your single evening snack. Turn off the light. If your kitchen has a door, close that, too. You can even put a sign on your kitchen counter: "See you at breakfast."

✦ Signal an end to the evening. Have a cup of tea, brush your teeth, gargle, read a book to your kids. Do whatever it is that means the evening (and snacking) is over.

SHARON O'S STORY

" Balancing my diet has dramatically decreased my cravings for sugar. I used to eat large quantities of desserts. I love chocolate and sweets! If I ate one cookie, I usually had to have at least four. Cakes, pies, ice cream—you name it, and I craved it. Now I'll only eat a bite of my husband's dessert. He gets to have his dessert and not feel guilty about eating it in front of me. Since I have a better diet, one bite satisfies my cravings. I still eat ice cream in the evenings, but a MUCH smaller portion, and I don't have a problem with that. "

Evening Snack

Limit yourself to one evening snack of 100–200 calories. The amount of carbohydrate you should eat is individualized based on your meal plan, blood glucose, and medications. For many people, up to 20 grams of carbohydrate before bed is appropriate. To limit temptation, tack up a list of suitable snacks somewhere in your kitchen. Choose only from that list. Here are a few ideas to get you started.

✦ ½ cup 2% cottage cheese with ¼ teaspoon vanilla extract and ground cinnamon to taste
Calories: 90   Carbs: 6

- 3 cups air-popped popcorn spritzed with butter spray and sprinkled with 1 tablespoon Parmesan cheese
  Calories: 120   Carbs: 19
- ½ cup fat-free ready-to-eat pudding
  Calories: 105   Carbs: 23
- ½ cup nonfat Greek yogurt mixed with ¼ cup applesauce (no sugar added) and ground cinnamon to taste
  Calories: 85   Carbs: 11
- 1 small apple, diced, and mixed with 1 tablespoon chopped walnuts, 2 tablespoons nonfat Greek yogurt, and sweetener to taste
  Calories: 140   Carbs: 22

RESET YOUR ROUTINE

Changing your routine to break a snack habit works at times other than bedtime. What things or events trigger you to overeat? Do you grab a snack from the mini-mart when you fill the gas tank or do you stop for a warm-from-the-oven donut on your way to work? Think through your week and use your food record to identify your triggers. Then set out to change them. For example, buy gas at a station that doesn't have a mini mart. Drive a couple of blocks out of your way to avoid the donut shop. Even entering the house through a different door has helped some people avoid raiding the refrigerator after work. Be creative.

REVISIT YOUR FOOD RECORD

Has writing down every sip and morsel of food for seven weeks gotten old? Remember, dieters who keep food records lose more weight than those who don't. Even though they recognize the value of a food record, a lot of people struggle to keep it up because writing everything down becomes a tedious, annoying task. Self-monitoring is critical for assessing your strengths and weaknesses and to re-strategize when things don't go right, but you do have a few options if you're tired of the traditional record. Below are a few approaches. If you're ready for a change, pick one and try it out. Turn to the Appendix for templates.

- **Trouble Times and Places.** Keep the same format, but write down only those times and places that require you to be the most vigilant. Some people choose to write down their dinner and nighttime snacks, but feel they have a good handle on other times of the day. Others record what they eat at work or all snacks or restaurant foods or their food choices at the mall or at parties. Record what's most problematic for you.

✦ **Trouble Foods.** If you eat too many sweets and not enough vegetables, record just sweets and vegetables.

✦ **Check It.** Select as many as five goals, such as eat breakfast and walk at lunchtime. Record your progress on a checklist.

✦ **Score It.** At the end of the day, write down a number between 1 and 10 to describe your success with specific goals, such as eating appropriate portions or planning your intake ahead. These are subjective scores for fairly vague goals. Though this format has value, it's better to make specific goals with easily measured, objective outcomes.

WEEK 7 ACTION STEPS

Continue your current goals or rewrite them if necessary. Additionally, select from the following goals or steps, modify them, or create your own. Choose goals from the previous weeks if applicable. This week I will:

☐ Continue the following goals: _____

_____

_____

☐ Eat breakfast daily.

☐ Write a list of acceptable snacks from which to choose.

☐ Avoid my trigger to overeat by doing the following _____.

☐ Start a ritual to signal the end of the evening _____.

☐ Continue my daily food record.

☐ Experiment with a new way to self-monitor my progress.

☐ Other: _____

Week

8

You've got a lot of the weight-loss basics down now. This week's tips cover hunger and restaurant meals and will enhance those basic skills.

KNOW YOUR HUNGER

Watching food commercials on television makes some people reach for snacks. The sight, smell, and even the thought of food might your trigger appetite. Some people eat out of habit or boredom, out of sadness or happiness. And for many people, years of both dieting and overeating have confused their sense of hunger, and they no longer recognize what true hunger is. If any of this describes you, use the ruler on the next page to identify your feelings of being hungry and full. Do this before and after your meals, and record the number in your food journal. Try to start your meal at level 3 or 4 (which are indicated) when you are hungry but not ravenous, and stop at 6 (also indicated) when your body has had just enough. Some people like to record their hunger for every hour that they are awake for just a few days to quickly get in touch with their body's hunger cues.

Hunger Ruler

1	2	3	4	5	6	7	8	9	10

1. starving, irritable, being this hungry is painful
2. very hungry, loud rumblings in your stomach
3. hungry, wanting to eat
4. just starting to get hungry
5. neither hungry nor full
6. just at that point of fullness, perfectly content

7. just beyond fullness; you've had enough but could find room for a few more bites
8. uncomfortable, wish you hadn't had those last few bites
9. very uncomfortable, bloated
10. so full that it feels like Thanksgiving

These exercises will help you become more mindful of eating. It should discourage you from eating at inappropriate times and encourage you to eat at the right times. Now keep in mind, however, that sometimes it's okay to eat when you're not hungry; say, when you're at a level 5. You might eat anyway to keep to your schedule, avoid being famished later, or maybe just because it's a special occasion.

FILL UP ON FIBER

Not only is fiber good for digestion, it can also help you lose weight by taming your hunger. Fruits, vegetables, whole grains, and beans are naturally high in fiber and should be your first choice for fiber-rich foods. Foods like breads and yogurts with added fibers are fine too, but let the naturally fiber-rich foods play a bigger role in your diet. If you make one part of your meal a good source of protein, like chicken or fish, and at least one part a good source of fiber (a good source of fiber has 2.5 grams of fiber per serving but 4–5 grams is even better), like broccoli or whole-grain pasta, you will be better able to control hunger. There's no need to fret over how many grams of fiber you eat each day. As long as you choose a variety of wholesome foods and eat adequate fruits, vegetables, and whole grains, you should be just fine. In general, however, the recommendations range from 21 to 38 grams fiber per day.

FIBER IN YOUR FOOD

Food	Serving Size/Exchange/ Food Choice*	Total Dietary Fiber (grams)
Apple, raw with skin	1 small fruit (1 Fruit)	3.6
Banana	1 medium fruit (1 Fruit)	3.1
Blueberries	¾ cup (1 Fruit)	2.7
Grapefruit	½ fruit (1 Fruit)	2.0
Orange, navel	1 fruit (1 Fruit)	3.1

Food	Serving Size/Exchange/Food Choice*	Total Dietary Fiber (grams)
Strawberries	1 ¼ cup, whole (1 Fruit)	3.6
Tomato	1 medium fruit (1 Nonstarchy Vegetable)	1.5
Oatmeal	½ cup cooked (1 Starch)	2.0
Corn flakes	¾ cup (1 Starch) 1 cup (1⅓ Starch)	0.5 0.7
Bran flakes	½ cup (1 Starch) 1 cup (2 Starch)	3.5 7.0
Grits	½ cup cooked (1 Starch) 1 cup cooked (2 Starch)	1.2 2.4
Shredded wheat cereal	½ cup (1 Starch) 1 cup (2 Starch)	2.5 5.0
Barley	⅓ cup cooked (1 Starch) 1 cup cooked (3 Starch)	2.0 6.0
Rice, white, long-grain, enriched	⅓ cup cooked (1 Starch) 1 cup cooked (3 Starch)	Less than 1 Less than 1
Rice, brown, long-grain	⅓ cup cooked (1 Starch) 1 cup cooked (3 Starch)	1.2 3.5
Quinoa	⅓ cup cooked (1 Starch) 1 cup cooked (3 Starch)	1.7 5.2
Spaghetti noodles, whole wheat	⅓ cup cooked (1 Starch) 1 cup cooked (3 Starch)	2.1 6.3
Spaghetti noodles, enriched	⅓ cup cooked (1 Starch) 1 cup cooked (3 Starch)	Less than 1 2.5
Broccoli	1 cup chopped, cooked (2 Nonstarchy Vegetable)	5.5
Green beans	1 cup cooked (2 Nonstarchy Vegetable)	4.0
Frozen corn kernels, yellow	½ cup (1 Starch) 1 cup (2 Starch)	1.8 3.7
Baby carrots, raw	7 medium carrots (1 Nonstarchy Vegetable)	2.0
Spinach	1 cup raw (Free Food)	0.7
Baked beans	⅓ cup (1 Starch) 1 cup (3 Starch)	3.2 9.6
Lima beans	½ cup (1 Starch) 1 cup (2 Starch)	5.4 10.8
Kidney beans	½ cup (1 Starch) 1 cup (2 Starch)	5.7 11.4
Green peas	½ cup (1 Starch) 1 cup (2 Starch)	4.4 8.8
Pretzels, plain	¾ oz (1 Starch)	0.6

Source: USDA Nutrient Data Laboratory (http://www.nal.usda.gov/fnic/foodcomp/search/index.html)

*Exchanges/Food Choices are a meal-planning tool designed to help people with diabetes develop and manage their meal plan. If you'd like to learn more about this tool, pick up a copy of *Choose Your Foods: Exchange Lists for Diabetes,* published by the American Diabetes Association.

EAT OUT

This week, take on a new challenge: go out to eat at a restaurant! Restaurant meals can be calorie bombs disguised as a healthful salad or saturated-fat land-mines masquerading as a wholesome wrap or sub sandwich. It's hard to tell what has been sautéed in gobs of butter or topped with sauces sweetened with obscene amounts of sugar. Portions are oversized and partly to blame for over-sized Americans. In many restaurants, the typical portion of food shows no resemblance to a reasonable amount.

Practice these strategies to keep calories down and nutritional quality up. Unfortunately, the sodium in restaurant food is almost always sky high.

1. **Preview the menu.** Look at the menu online or stop by the restaurant a few minutes early to decide which are your best choices. If possible, know what you're going to order before you even walk through the door.

2. **Be pushy.** Be the first to order, so you're not influenced by the choices of your dining companions. Ask lots of questions about food preparation, and make special requests for foods prepared with less fat, salt, and added sugars. Ask that the staff not bring bread or chips. If someone else at the table wants them, push the basket out of your reach.

3. **Order smart.** Fill up on fewer calories. Ask for double vegetables, and start your meal with a low-calorie salad or a broth-based soup. Under-stand that these menu descriptors usually mean that the food is high in calories, fat, or, most frequently, both calories and fat: *crispy, batter-dipped, basted, deep-fried, coated, marinated, creamy, rich, Alfredo.* Ask for the food to be prepared differently or choose another item off the menu.

4. **Be picky.** Don't use up your calorie or carbohydrate budget on food that isn't delicious. If it isn't awesome, push it aside. At a buffet, scrutinize the array of food before selecting any, and use a salad plate instead of a dinner plate.

5. **Don't drink your calories.** Regular sodas, sweetened tea, and alcohol load on the calories without filling you up. Stick to water. If indulging in alcohol, limit yourself to just one drink.

6. **Pay attention to your food.** It's easy to overeat when you're distracted by conversation. Focus on every bite and every sip. Take close notice of your food. How does it look? What is the texture? The aroma? Look at it and savor it.

7. **Slow down.** Instead of keeping up with the fastest eater at the table, pace yourself with the slowest person or plan to be that slowest eater. Try to be the last person to start eating.

8. **Keep tabs on portions.** Just know that whatever you're served is likely way more than you need, so plan from the start to leave food on your plate. You have several options:
   - Decide on your proper portion. Then draw an imaginary line through your food, and don't cross that line.
   - When you place your order, ask to have half of your meal boxed to go.
   - Order an appetizer, half portion, or a lunch portion, which are usually smaller and less expensive than the dinner portion.
   - Share with a friend.

9. **Reconsider the meaning of value.** Some diners are most influenced by cost and order the least expensive items on the menu. Some eat more if the food is expensive, so they can "get their money's worth." Instead of letting cost rule, pay attention to health value and nutritional value. If cost is a major factor, choose the least expensive healthful choice or share something with a companion. Instead of feeling wasteful for leaving food, remind yourself that if your body doesn't need it, you're wasting it whether you eat it or leave it. It's better to leave it behind.

WHAT TO EAT WHEN EATING OUT

Use this guide to make the best choices in any type of restaurant.

Asian

GO FOR IT:

- Steamed dumplings, steamed spring roll
- Miso, wonton, egg drop, and hot and sour soups: these tend to be low in calories, but be aware that your cup is probably spilling over with sodium
- Veggie-heavy dishes: moo goo gai pan, steamed fish with vegetables, and stir-fried meat or tofu and vegetables
- Use chopsticks: they'll slow you down and help you drain some of the fat- and sodium-drenched sauces
- Hot tea: unsweetened, of course

- Fortune cookie: for a mere 30 calories and 7 grams of carbohydrate, think of all the fun these little cookies provide

USE CAUTION:

- Buffets, fast-food, and mall fare: meats are often fried and reheated in extra oil
- General Tso's chicken: outrageous calories and saturated fat because the meat is fried
- Sweet and sour entrées: more fried meats here, plus sugar-laden sauce
- Chow mein: fried noodles
- Other fried foods: crispy noodles (soup topping), fried rice, egg rolls, shrimp toast

Italian

GO FOR IT:

- Minestrone and bean soups
- House salad: ask for the dressing on the side
- Prosciutto with melon
- Tomato-based sauces without cream or fatty meats over pasta, fish, or chicken: tomato, pomodoro, marinara, red clam, puttanesca

USE CAUTION:

- Eggplant, veal, and chicken Parmesan: floured, fried, and heavy on cheese
- Lasagna and other baked casseroles: too much cheese and usually made with fatty meats
- Alfredo sauce: a mix of butter, cream, and Parmesan cheese
- Carbonara sauce: rich in fat from eggs, cream, cheese, and Italian bacon

Mexican

GO FOR IT:

- Black bean soup
- Tortilla soup: hold the bacon and limit the cheese and fried tortilla chips
- Salsa and picante sauce: skip the fried chips. Instead use salsa and picante sauce to dress your salad and to spice up tacos, soups, and more

- Guacamole: contains healthful fats, just limit your portion
- Arroz con pollo: chicken and rice
- Soft tacos: limit the cheese and sour cream
- Fajitas: request that the sizzling oil or butter be left off your plate

USE CAUTION:

- Crispy tortillas: these are fried
- Chimichanga: a deep-fried burrito
- Salad shells: deep-fried, often about 500 calories alone, before you fill them
- Chili rellenos: deep-fried stuffed peppers
- Refried beans: ask your server if these are made with unhealthful lard. If not, go for it.

Middle Eastern

GO FOR IT:

- Hummus: dip or spread made with chickpeas
- Lentil soup: great source of fiber
- Cucumber-yogurt soup: if made with reduced-fat yogurt
- Tabbouleh: salad of cracked wheat, tomatoes, parsley, and more
- Greek salad: go easy on the dressing
- Shish kebobs

USE CAUTION:

- Falafel: fried bean patty
- Spanakopita: phyllo dough filled with spinach and feta cheese
- Pasticcio: casserole of ground beef and macaroni in a creamy sauce
- Moussaka: casserole of eggplant and meat in a cheesy-creamy sauce

American Fare and Fast Food

GO FOR IT:

- Scooped bagel: fewer calories and carbs because the doughiest part is scooped out
- Sandwiches with lean meats, such as roast beef, turkey, and chicken. Fatten up your sandwich with extra veggies, not extra meats and cheese

- Salads with lots of colorful veggies, a little dressing, and not much of anything else
- Lean entrées without creamy or buttery sauces: try steamed shrimp, grilled tuna, baked salmon, sirloin steak, baked chicken (without the skin)
- Rotisserie chicken without skin
- Steamed vegetables
- Fast-food sandwich from the children's menu: built-in portion control

USE CAUTION:

- Croissants and biscuits: prepared with lots of fat
- Broccoli-cheese soup, cream of potato soup, and other creamy or cheesy soups
- Deep-fried sides like French fries and onion rings
- Fried chicken or fried fish
- Fatty meats such as prime rib, beef or pork ribs, corned beef, chicken with skin, sausage, bacon, and hot dogs
- Large or super-sized sandwiches or burgers
- Turkey burgers: frequently includes ground turkey skin
- Chicken salad, egg salad, tuna salad: extra calories from the mayonnaise
- Sauces and dressings such as cheese, béarnaise, and hollandaise sauces, mayonnaise, gravy, and salad dressings: use very little because of the high calories and high saturated fat content

FOR MORE INFORMATION

Websites

American Cancer Society:
www.cancer.org/Healthy/EatHealthyGetActive/TakeControlofYourWeight/restaurant-eating-tips (provides ordering tips and fast-food information)

American Diabetes Association:
www.diabetes.org/food-and-fitness/food/what-can-i-eat/eating-out/ (discusses the timing of diabetes medications when eating out and how to find hidden fats)

Cooperative Extension System:
www.extension.org/pages/24398/interactive-fast-food-menu (an interactive fast-food menu)

Healthy Dining Finder:

www.healthydiningfinder.com (identifies restaurants and menu items that meet specific nutrition criteria)

National Restaurant Association:

www.restaurant.org/foodhealthyliving/foodenthusiasts/eatingsmart (provides ordering tips for trimming calories and boosting nutrition)

Books

Guide to Healthy Restaurant Eating: What to eat in America's most popular chain restaurants, 4th ed. by Hope S. Warshaw, MMSC, RD, CDE, BC-ADM (American Diabetes Association, 2009)

Eat Out Healthy, by Joanne V. Lichten, PhD, RD (Nutrifit Publishing, 2012)

Guide to Healthy Fast Food Eating, 2nd ed. by Hope S. Warshaw, MMSC, RD, CDE, BC-ADM (American Diabetes Association, 2009)

Restaurant Calorie Counter for Dummies by Roseanne Rust, MS, RD, LDN, and Meri Raffetto, RD (John Wiley & Sons, Inc., 2011)

MARCIA C'S STORY

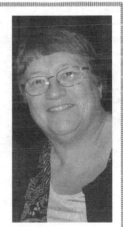

❝ We probably eat out five or six times a week. I've learned a lot of strategies over the years that are still helpful: eat smaller portions, cut food into small pieces, put fork down between bites, and box half the entrée for the next day. I also get hot tea or coffee and a glass of water. If the menu isn't diet friendly, I ask how it could be made better. Can I get fruit, cottage cheese, or tomatoes instead of toast or home fries? I ask for double the vegetable portion, dressings and gravies on the side, and no bread. If my husband wants bread, I ask that they bring it only to him. I'm not shy about telling the waiter or waitress that I have diabetes and need to make wise choices. Most of the time they're anxious to help and it eliminates the hard sell on tasty but deadly desserts. ❞

WEEK 8 ACTION STEPS

Continue your current goals or rewrite them if necessary. Additionally, select from the following goals or steps, modify them, or create your own. Choose goals from the previous weeks if applicable. This week I will:

☐ Continue the following goals: _____

_____

_____

☐ Use the Hunger Ruler before and after at least one meal each day.

☐ Try to end each meal before I am overfull.

☐ Eat at least two foods that are good sources of fiber at each meal.

☐ Get more fiber by _____ .

☐ Use a restaurant guide when eating out.

☐ Use the Internet and books to find nutrition information for restaurant food.

☐ Be the slowest eater at the table for every meal.

☐ Be more active by _____ .

Week 9

You've been at this for two months now. You probably have some strategies and skills down very well, others maybe not so well. You may have even found that some things that were easy a few weeks ago are no longer easy. That's typical, and that's why we revisit similar topics in new ways. Here we take another look at portion control, preparing your own food, and being physically active.

SIZE MATTERS

Limiting your portions might be one of your most important strategies to lose weight. When researchers studied the effects of controlling portions, limiting fat intake, eating more fruits and vegetables, and getting more physical activity, they found that the dieters who spent more time and effort practicing portion control lost the most weight. Most people will need to do all or most of these things (and more) to lose weight or even to keep from gaining weight, but this study is a good reminder that eating small portions of treats now and then is okay.

If you routinely eat more than your body needs or wants, try a few of these portion-control strategies.

- ✦ House Rule: No eating unless the food is in a dish. This means no digging your hand into the box of crackers, bag of candy, or even taking a few bites from someone else's plate. Everything has to be in your own dish.
- ✦ If you didn't pre-portion your chips and crackers in Week 5, do it this week. Pre-measure crackers, chips, nuts, cookies, and other tempting or high-calorie foods into individual baggies or containers. Store them all

in the original packaging. Grab one for a snack or as an addition to your meal.

- ✦ Eating Out Rule: No super-sizing and no meal deals.
- ✦ Fill your bowls, cups, and glasses with water. Then pour the water into a measuring cup to see how big the dish is. Now you have a way to estimate your food without pulling out measuring cups each time.
- ✦ Use a baby spoon or espresso spoon to make ice cream, pudding, yogurt, and other spoonable treats last longer.
- ✦ Pre-plate your meal using the Plate Method (see Week 2). Or, serve meats and starches from the kitchen. Put leftovers away before you even take your first bite of food. Serve nonstarchy vegetables at the table to make second helpings of veggies easy.
- ✦ Eat low-calorie nonstarchy vegetables before serving yourself other foods.
- ✦ Try a few low-calorie, portion-controlled, frozen or shelf-stable meals to help you relearn or visualize appropriate portions. Add a salad, some nonstarchy vegetables, or both to give you better nutrition and help you feel full longer.
- ✦ Take a fast course in portions: weigh and measure everything you eat and drink for five days.
- ✦ Slow down. Put your fork down between bites. Sip water frequently. Time your meals and try to make them last 30 minutes. Here's a silly one, but it works: when eating alone, watch yourself in the mirror to see how quickly you eat.
- ✦ Wear something just a little snug around the waist to remind you not to overeat.
- ✦ Take the National Heart, Lung, and Blood Institute's Portion Distortion Quiz online (hp2010.nhlbihin.net/portion).

COOL TOOLS FOR PROPER PORTIONS
Fight portion distortion with these handy tools.

- ▮ **Food Scales:** You have lots of options here. Choose a model that simply weighs your food or a fancy one that provides information on calories, carbohydrates, sodium, and more. You can even find accurate scales so tiny that they fit in the palm of your hand and are perfect for taking to work and restaurants.

- **Measuring Cups:** These are an absolute must-have. Buy a standard set consisting of ¼-cup, ⅓-cup, ½-cup, and 1-cup measures. Additional sizes such as ⅛-cup and 2-cup measures are also handy, but less critical. If you're short on space, consider a set of collapsible measuring cups.
- **Portion Plates:** You won't need measuring cups or a food scale at dinner if you use a portion plate. Some are simple divided plates with different sections for meat, starches, and vegetables. Others have pictures of food that indicate where you are to place each type of food. Others indicate the proper portions but it is hidden within a stylish design. For example, place your vegetables over the largest flower and meat over the smallest. Search for "portion plate" on the Internet to find many options.

MORE FROM BARBARA C.

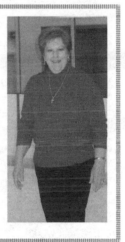

❝ I still weigh and measure my food—even after losing about 40 pounds and keeping it off for three years. It's one of the things that helps me keep tabs on how much I eat. I also freeze food in the portions that I'm going to eat them, and I even weigh out dry pasta to cook just one serving at a time. Before, I was never able to maintain the weight I lost. Now I weigh 10 pounds less than when I got married! ❞

PACK A SACK

Making lunch at home, whether you travel to work or not, is a smart strategy to limit calories and manage blood pressure, blood glucose, and cholesterol. A typical fast food or casual restaurant meal saddles you with at least half the calories that an average adult should have for the whole day. The numbers for saturated fat and sodium are even scarier, and low-carb options often have the most calories, sodium, and unhealthy fats.

Turn packing lunch into a habit. If you like leftovers, prepare your lunch while cleaning up after dinner. If you prefer a sandwich or a frozen meal or anything else, get it ready the night before, so running late in the morning doesn't mean no lunch. Even if you eat at home, preparing your lunch the night before can help you stick to your plan. If you carry your lunch to work, have an insulated lunch bag, some cold packs, and storage containers and bags of various sizes. Some people like to use portion plates with lids. If friends at work like to pack healthful lunches, too, take turns making lunches and trying new recipes.

Make lunch something to look forward to. Get creative and go for variety. Try a sandwich with almond butter and sliced apples or a wrap with roast beef, onion, roasted red peppers, and horseradish sauce. How about a spinach salad with egg, onion, beets, and chopped nuts or leftover rice mixed with diced ham, chopped bell peppers, black olives, sun-dried tomatoes, and low-calorie salad dressing? Mix and match these for a fun, innovative lunch entrée.

Base	Filling/Protein	Veggies	Condiments
Mixed lettuce	Almond or peanut butter	Beets	Chopped nuts
Baby spinach	Sliced egg	Cucumber	Thinly sliced apples or pears
100% whole-wheat bread	Tuna salad (with low-fat mayonnaise)	Tomato	Fresh basil, cilantro, or dill
100% whole-wheat tortilla	Hummus	Onion	Mustard
Whole-grain crackers	Canned beans, mashed or whole	Lettuce	Reduced-fat mayonnaise
Whole-rye bread	Roast beef	Baby spinach leaves	Horseradish sauce (low fat)
100% whole-wheat sandwich roll	Sliced turkey or chicken	Bell peppers (red, yellow, orange, green)	Reduced-fat ranch dressing or other favorite dressing
100% whole-wheat pita	Rotisserie chicken	Avocado	Guacamole
Leftover rice, pasta, or quinoa	Smoked turkey breast	Jarred roasted red peppers	Hummus
	Ham	Sun-dried tomatoes	BBQ sauce
	Leftover grilled shrimp	Snow peas	Salsa
	Reduced-fat cheese	Black olives	Mango chutney
	Leftover baked or grilled salmon	Sliced mushrooms	Feta or blue cheese crumbles

Round out your lunch with one or more of the following: soup, yogurt, side salad, chopped salad or slaw, bean salad, fruit, crackers, nuts, or nonfat milk.

MORE FROM FRANK P.

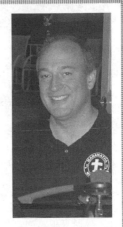

66 I now make my lunch most days. It helps me to eat better and save money at the same time. In my line of work, it's often difficult to break free for lunch, so packing it helps me avoid missing a meal. Making it the night before or in the morning is extra work, but worth it. It means I have to plan ahead to keep the right foods, such as vegetables, rye bread, yogurt, and fruit, in the house. One of my favorites is a whole-wheat wrap that I make with grilled chicken, vegetables, beans, and low-fat or nonfat cheese. I also make sandwiches with rye bread or whole-wheat flatbread. I like frozen peas and carrots, stir-fry vegetable mix, or broccoli and cauliflower mix. I fill a container with a cup or two of frozen vegetables and let them thaw at my desk. They're great at room temperature or slightly cold for lunch. My all-time favorite, however, is my fiber cereal snack. I use Fiber One cereal, All Bran cereal, or raw oats, or all three, and add cinnamon, nuts, and a tablespoon of chocolate morsels. At lunch, I mix some of it with nonfat Greek yogurt and save the rest for an afternoon snack.

Changing the foods I eat has another benefit. It seems like when I eat heathy, the food tastes better. For example, if I have fresh vegetables piled onto a sandwich with only a slice or two of meat (instead of all meat and cheese) and if I don't add any salt and instead season it with only the basics, like balsamic vinegar and a dash of olive oil or Dijon mustard, that's a great meal. It's like night and day compared to the way I was eating before—a more memorable event when the difference in taste is realized. 99

CHECKING IN WITH EXERCISE

How is the exercise going? If you're wearing a pedometer, your step count should be a good bit higher than when you started several weeks ago. If you're recording your activity level, you can compare what you're doing now with your activity level in Week 1. If you're not as active as you think you should be, ask yourself why. Have you made SMART exercise goals and worked at them? Have you made it a priority? Use the Motivation and Confidence Ruler from Week 5 (page 46) and review SMART goal setting in the Introduction (page 4) to move yourself along.

Sometimes people get discouraged because they think the exercise recommendations are out of reach. Don't let that stop you. Remember that getting any exercise is better than none. Do what is reasonable for you now. You can always reevaluate later.

LISA M'S STORY

" I used to think that I didn't have enough time to exercise with my busy schedule. Then, I just decided that exercise had to become part of my day, so I moved some of the other things around until I fit it in. I started walking around the block once, which is half of a mile. Then, after about a week, I walked around the block twice a day. Now I use weights two or three times a week, too. Sometimes the dishes sit a little longer or the laundry waits to be folded, but that's okay. "

WEEK 9 ACTION STEPS

Continue your current goals or rewrite them if necessary. Additionally, select from the following goals or steps, modify them, or create your own. Choose goals from the previous weeks if applicable. This week I will:

☐ Continue the following goals: _____

_____

_____

☐ Eat only when sitting at the table and when eating from a dish.

☐ Serve meats and starches from the kitchen, but keep vegetables on the table.

☐ Weigh and measure the following foods_____

_____

_____.

☐ Use a food scale.

☐ Continue using my food record or alternative form of self-monitoring.

☐ Pack lunch at least three times.

☐ Purchase the following so I can make a balanced lunch: _____

_____

_____.

☐ Add 10 minutes to my usual walk at least twice.

☐ Other: _____

Week 10

Losing weight and keeping it off requires that you have skills for all types of situations. Up until now, we've focused on your average day. This week, we take a look at handling weekends, vacations, and special occasions. We'll continue this discussion next week, when we address sticking to your diet plan while at parties. But first, here's one more way to use veggies to keep you full and satisfied.

BULK UP YOUR MEALS

Do you want more meatloaf, macaroni and cheese, or potato salad than your waistline and blood glucose should have? Sometimes just a half cup of a favorite food is just right, but other times, it's terribly unsatisfying. Don't fret, though. Here are some tactics that will help you out.

In Week 6, you learned to swap one ingredient for another to lower the fat and calories in your recipes. This week, you'll work on making your portion bigger without increasing the calories and carbs. By slipping in some vegetables, you can actually eat more for less. For example, instead of having one-half cup traditional mac and cheese, enjoy a full cup of reduced-fat mac and cheese with tomatoes and broccoli. Also, consider hiding puréed vegetables in your casseroles, soups, and baked goods. When researchers at Pennsylvania State University did this, the men and women eating in the research lab cut their daily intake by about 350 calories. The bonus? More vegetables and better nutrition.

Try these vegetable sneaks:

✦ Replace some lasagna noodles with very thinly sliced zucchini. A mandolin is a kitchen tool that thinly slices ingredients, and having one can be very helpful with this. Look for a mandolin in kitchen stores.

- Add lightly steamed or thawed frozen broccoli and canned tomatoes to macaroni and cheese. Be sure to use reduced-fat cheese.
- Tuck puréed broccoli or carrots into tomato-based casseroles.
- Layer sautéed mushrooms and onions over the cheese in a tortilla.
- Give a grilled cheese sandwich a lift with sliced tomato and fresh basil leaves.
- Chop colorful bell peppers, celery, and red onion for both tuna salad and pasta salad. Grape tomatoes and sugar snap peas also work well with pasta salad.
- Add a bag of thawed frozen vegetables to pasta salad. Choose your favorite veggie combination or whatever is on sale.
- Give potato salad some color with steamed, chopped green beans, roasted beets, or other favorite veggies.
- Turn plain rice fancy by adding diced and sautéed summer squash, asparagus, onions, celery, and herbs.
- Top spaghetti squash instead of pasta with your favorite sauce.
- Chop Portobello mushrooms and toss with any beef dish. Portobellos have a very meaty flavor.
- Mix grated zucchini or carrots or puréed vegetables into ground meat for meatloaf or meatballs.
- Substitute puréed cauliflower for half the potatoes in mashed potatoes.
- Make a veggie omelet instead of one with ham and cheese.
- See the Appendix (page 198) for three bulked-up recipes: Judy's Lightened Meatloaf, Veggie-Packed Potato Salad, and Rita's New England Clam Chowder.

RECIPE TIP!

Melissa Nodvin, MS, RD, substitutes puréed butternut squash for part of the cheese in her version of lightened macaroni and cheese. For a mild squash taste, replace about 25% of the cheese with squash. If you want a stronger taste of the vegetable, use as much as one-third squash to two-thirds cheese sauce. For speed and simplicity, buy frozen butternut squash that has been already puréed. To purée fresh squash, cut it into chunks and add a little water or low-sodium vegetable stock. Place in a blender or food processor and process until smooth.

STAY THE COURSE
ON THE WEEKENDS

TGIF! Who doesn't look forward to the weekend, vacations, and special events? It's important to enjoy time off without extra food, however. It's much too easy to undo all of your hard work from the week before. Researchers with the National Weight Control Registry (see Week 3 and Month 12 for more information about the NWCR), a registry of over 5,000 people who have lost at least 30 pounds and kept it off for at least one year, learned that day-to-day consistency is important for maintaining weight loss. Loosening up the diet plan on the weekends or special occasions is such a common tendency and one that's easy to ignore or rationalize away. Special meals out can easily have more than 1,500 calories. Add dessert and a drink or two, and you're hitting more than 2,000 calories—all in one meal! Throw in some mall fare earlier in the day and your calories are sky high. Even a fancy burger in a casual restaurant can saddle you with more than 1,000 calories—and that's not including fries or other sides.

Some people nibble all weekend when they're home. Some sleep late and skip exercise. Some people just plain lose focus on the weekends or when they're away from home because they're more relaxed. So how can you keep the same vigilance on the weekends or on vacations that you have at other times? Be sure you try to stick to a schedule, even if it's not the same schedule you have during the week. Eat breakfast, have lunch a few hours later, and dinner a few hours after that. Find time for exercise, even if it's different from your usual routine, and make tradeoffs. If you want spaghetti at your favorite Italian restaurant, skip the bread and drinks and take an extra walk. Keep a detailed food record. Even if you use a shorter food record during the week or no food record at all (and this is a good time to remind you that food records work!), track your intake in as much detail as possible over the weekend. Don't forget to remind yourself of your goals. If you falter, pick yourself back up and get back on track, and don't try to be perfect. A perfect diet doesn't exist, and trying to behave that way has sent many dieters into a binge.

HENRY S'S STORY

"Everything about dieting and diabetes is a challenge. One thing that's especially hard for me is eating healthfully when I go out to dinner and to the ballet. The biggest thing for success is consistency, so I try to eat in places that have broiled fish and other healthy food. I've already figured out what I have to do, and now I've got to stick with it. If I deviate, I go right back to it. I can't say all is lost and then go hog wild. I go back to it, and I even cut back a little too. I should have done it this way years ago."

TO DRINK OR NOT TO DRINK?

The decision to drink alcohol is between you and your doctor. Among other things, that decision will depend on your calorie needs, blood glucose control, and medications. If you decide to drink, pay special attention to your blood glucose. Alcohol can cause hypoglycemia shortly after drinking, or it can even occur the following day because the liver is unable to release glucose into the bloodstream. You are especially at risk for hypoglycemia if you take medications that have that as a potential side effect (namely, insulin, sulfonylureas, and meglitinides). If you're unsure if you take any of these medications, call your pharmacist or doctor's office. Lessen the risk of having low blood glucose by eating pretzels, bread, fruit, or other food containing carbohydrate while you drink. You might also experience high blood glucose when drinking, but that is not from the alcohol. High blood glucose occurs from the food you eat at the same time or from the carbohydrate-containing beverage you mix with your drink.

Alcoholic drinks also have calories that you must consider. If you cut back on food to save calories, you'll be even more likely to experience hypoglycemia. But if you don't cut calories, you won't be able to lose weight. It is best to follow your usual meal plan when drinking alcoholic beverages and to drink only a moderate amount (see next page). Additionally, measure blood glucose more often when you drink alcohol to see how it affects you. Measure it an hour or two after drinking, before driving, at bedtime, and even more often, including the middle of the night, if you are unsure how your blood glucose is reacting.

What Is Moderate Drinking?

Because women metabolize alcohol more slowly than men, the definition of "moderate drinking" is different for the sexes. For men, moderate drinking is having no more than two drinks per day. For women, it's having no more than one drink daily. One drink is

- ✦ 1 bottle or can (12 fluid ounces) of beer
- ✦ 1.5 fluid ounces of 80-proof liquor such as bourbon and vodka
- ✦ 1 fluid ounce of 100-proof liquor such as bourbon and vodka
- ✦ 4–5 fluid ounces of wine

CALORIE COUNTS OF COMMON ALCOHOLIC BEVERAGES

Beverage	Calories	Carbohydrate (g)
Beer, 12 fluid ounces	120–180	9–16
Light Beer, 12 fluid ounces	70–110	3–8
Wine, 4 fluid ounces	80–100	2–4
Bourbon, 1.5 fluid ounce 80-proof	100	0
Bourbon, 1 fluid ounce 100-proof	85	0
Piña Colada, 4.5 fluid ounces	245	32
8 fluid ounces	435	57

Being Moderate

It's tough to say no when you're out with friends, but limiting the amount you drink is important for your weight and blood glucose control.

- ✦ Sip slowly and avoid pressure from others to pick up the pace.
- ✦ Start your evening with a nonalcoholic drink like sparkling water with a twist of lime. For something more filling and with a little zip, try tomato or vegetable juice with lemon and a couple drops of hot sauce.
- ✦ Alternate alcoholic beverages with non-alcoholic ones. Drink at least as much water as alcoholic beverages.
- ✦ Keep track of how much you're drinking by refilling your own glass and avoiding topping off your drinks.
- ✦ Look for low-alcohol and non-alcoholic beers and wine.
- ✦ Make a wine spritzer. Mix equal parts wine with club soda or diet ginger ale.
- ✦ Wear medical ID when drinking.

WEEK 10 ACTION STEPS

Continue your current goals or rewrite them if necessary.
Additionally, select from the following goals or steps,
modify them, or create your own. Choose goals from the previous
weeks if applicable. This week I will:

☐ Continue the following goals: _____

_____

_____

☐ Try at least two strategies to add vegetables to my recipes.

☐ Eat at least three cups of nonstarchy vegetables every day.

☐ Keep a detailed food record on the weekends.

☐ Maintain my food record and eating plan while on vacation.

☐ Take a 30-minute walk Saturday and Sunday.

☐ Drink a low-calorie nonalcoholic beverage before drinking alcohol.

☐ Drink alcohol only on Friday or Saturday.

☐ Take my blood glucose meter with me when I'm planning to drink
away from home and use it.

☐ Other: _____

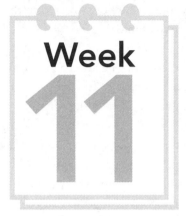

Week 11

We continue our look at handling special occasions this week. We'll also review your progress, examine additional food label traps, and discuss how a good night's sleep can help you manage both your weight and your diabetes.

IT'S PARTY TIME!

Whether it's a holiday, a birthday, or simply a bunch of friends enjoying the night together, parties have a way of weakening one's resolve. Some people avoid all parties, restaurants, and other situations that might cause them to overeat. While it's understandable to want to avoid temptation, it's not very realistic. It's far better to learn to deal with the situation, because it will come up again and again and again. Remember, we're working on building skills and strategies instead of relying on willpower. You can improve your chances of success in these situations by planning for them.

Party Strategies

Some of the following strategies have already been discussed in other sections of the book, but good ideas are worth repeating.

+ Before you even head out the door for the party, decide what tradeoffs you will make. You can eat *whatever* you want, but you cannot eat *everything* you want or *as much* as you want. You might be tempted by drinks before dinner and drinks during dinner, appetizers, bread, fried foods, dessert, or any number of things. Don't wait for the enticing aromas to decide for you. Before you get to the party, make a firm decision about what you will and will not eat. If you really want birthday cake, either satisfy yourself with just a bite or two or skip the bread, pasta, and other sweet and starchy foods.

+ Don't save up from breakfast and lunch to splurge at the party. Your friends without diabetes may be able to get away with this, but you cannot. The amount and type of food you eat at each snack and meal affects your blood glucose after eating. If you skimp early in the day and take certain diabetes medications, you risk having low blood glucose. If you overindulge after skipping meals, you risk high blood glucose.

+ Control your hunger (and your blood glucose) before the party. If the event is late or if you'll be eating dinner later than usual, have a snack before you go. A large glass of vegetable juice is very filling (only 70 calories and 15 grams of carbohydrate). Add some reduced-fat cheese to make your snack more substantial. You might also try a small apple with a tablespoon of peanut butter or dip some veggies and a few crackers into hummus. Eat just enough to take the edge off your appetite and keep your blood glucose steady.

+ Dance the night away. Be as active as possible before, during, and after the party. If you have just a few minutes to exercise, take a walk after eating. Researchers from Old Dominion University in Virginia found that walking for 20 minutes shortly after dinner lowered after-meal blood glucose more than a walk before eating.

+ If the food is served in a buffet, look over everything that's offered before selecting anything. Be very picky, and choose only one or two small splurges. Make your meal nutrient-dense and moderate in calories, carbohydrate, and saturated fat.

+ Start the evening with a low-calorie, non-alcoholic beverage, such as sparkling water or diet soda, and with filling, low-calorie food, such as steamed shrimp and raw vegetables.

+ Bring food to share, such as a vegetable tray or exotic fruit like figs and persimmons or strawberries dipped in chocolate.

+ When you've had enough to eat, position yourself far from the food and hold something in your hand, so you don't idly reach for food. If you usually have a shoulder bag, for example, carry a clutch to the party to keep your hands occupied.

+ Keep yourself occupied with conversation and other non-food activities.

+ Wear something that makes you look fabulous or something just a tad tight in the waist. Either will remind you to keep tabs on your intake.

YOUR PROGRESS REPORT

You've heard this many times before, but it's worth saying again because it is so, so important. Progress is much more than your weight or your dress size or your belt size. Look back at your early food and activity records. Think about your habits and even the way you thought about food and diet before you started this program more than two months ago. The number of changes you've made will probably surprise you. Use the Progress Report on page 181 in the Appendix to list your accomplishments. Include all medical improvements, like better glucose control and lower cholesterol, and every lifestyle change, like eating breakfast and taking the stairs at work. List positive changes in attitude and how you feel throughout your day. Ask close friends and family members what changes they have noticed. People close to you are likely aware of things that you haven't noticed. Take pride in each triumph, no matter how big or small. Add to this list often, and refer to it whenever you need a boost in motivation.

MICHAEL B'S STORY

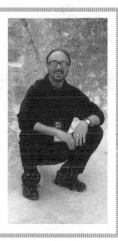

" Last year, when I would mow our hilly, land-scaped lawn, I had to do the 3 ½-hour job over two days. That's when I was 70 pounds heavier. Today I worked all morning on the school landscaping. Then, I came home to mow the lawn and completed it all in three hours. Afterward, I felt great! Losing weight has changed my health and changed my life. "

SUGAR-FREE FOODS

No doubt you've noticed a slew of sugar-free breads, cakes, pies, and candies in the supermarket. Some of these products have misleading labels. Remember that calories are the key to managing your weight, as carbohydrates are to your blood glucose. A sugar-free cookie, for example, may or may not be lower in calories or carbohydrates than the regular version of the food. Even if a cookie has no sugar, there are still carbohydrates from the flour. Sugar alcohols (which are carbohydrates), such as sorbitol and xylitol, may also be used to make the cookie sweet. These will affect blood glucose, although not as much as regular sugar. You will have to measure your blood glucose before and after eating them to see how a product with sugar alcohols (or any food) affects you. Just as you have learned in previous lessons, check the Nutrition Facts panel for the serving size, the calories, and total carbohydrates.

Just one more caution about sugar-free desserts: many, especially sugar-free ice creams, are very high in saturated fat, with as much as 5 grams of saturated fat per half cup. Because saturated fat affects your LDL cholesterol levels, eating products that are high in saturated fat is unwise, no matter how low they are in calories and carbohydrates.

HIT THE HAY

Which is most important: exercise, diet, or sleep? It's a trick question! None of the three is optional. When it comes to your health and well-being, all three are critical. In our "go, go, go" society, where we all have too much to do and too little time in which to do it, it's easy to sacrifice one or more of the three. For many, the first to go is sleep. Sleeping too little, however, affects hormone levels, impairs learning and memory, increases your risk of infection, and may even contribute to obesity, heart disease, and diabetes.

Research shows that individuals who sleep five or fewer hours each day, including naps, are twice as likely to have cardiovascular disease as those who sleep seven hours per day. Even one night of bad sleep affects blood glucose. Researchers in the Netherlands found that restricting sleep to four hours decreased insulin sensitivity by 20–25% compared with sleeping 8½ hours. Other research shows that sleep-deprived individuals snack more frequently and on more carbohydrate-rich foods. So you see, sleep really isn't optional if you want to control your weight and your overall health.

If good sleep seems like just a sweet dream, making a few simple changes may offer relief.

- ✦ Schedule a bedtime and do your best to stick with it.
- ✦ Relax prior to bedtime. Make it a ritual. Enjoy a cup of decaf or herbal tea, take a relaxing bath, read a book, listen to soothing music, meditate, or practice yoga. Avoid vigorous exercise and disturbing books, magazines, and television shows.
- ✦ Avoid caffeine, alcohol, and large meals several hours before bed.
- ✦ If frequent urination from high blood glucose is keeping you awake, call your doctor's office to see what changes you should make. If low blood glucose wakes you up, speak to your doctor immediately.
- ✦ If you are sleeping through the night but find yourself feeling tired in the morning, you could have a condition called sleep apnea. Sleep apnea

is characterized by periods of irregular breathing while sleeping and is common in people with diabetes. Talk to your doctor if you have trouble feeling well rested after sleep.

WEEK 11 ACTION STEPS

Continue your current goals or rewrite them if necessary. Additionally, select from the following goals or steps, modify them, or create your own. Choose goals from the previous weeks if applicable. This week I will:

☐ Continue the following goals: _____

_____

_____

☐ Be vigilant about reading food labels.

☐ Try at least one new recipe.

☐ Spend time with friends engaging in activities that do not revolve around eating or drinking.

☐ Complete my Progress Report. Ask my spouse/friend to fill it out with me.

☐ Track my fruit and vegetable intake on my food record.

☐ Plan to have a light snack if my meals will be late.

☐ Get to bed by 10:00 p.m. Sunday through Thursday.

☐ Allow myself at least 30 minutes to wind down before bedtime.

☐ Other: _____

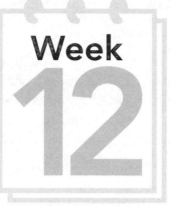

Week 12

Week 12 brings an in-depth look at eating between meals. You'll learn when to snack, what to snack on, and how to avoid inappropriate snacking by conquering your cravings and distracting yourself when necessary.

PUT SNACKS TO WORK

For most adults, even those with diabetes, snacks are optional. Research studies do not support the notion that eating frequently will help you lose weight or control your blood glucose any better than eating just breakfast, lunch, and dinner. In fact, some research suggests that men have better appetite control when they eat three larger meals per day compared with six smaller meals per day. (The research study didn't involve women.) For many people, snacking just means more calories overall. You should snack if you are hungry, to avoid becoming overly hungry later, to find an opportunity to eat important food groups that you'd miss otherwise, and *possibly* to avoid hypoglycemia. (If you have frequent hypoglycemia, you should talk to your doctor about changing your medications. You might need less medication or a different medication, especially if you've lost weight or are now exercising more.)

If snacks are right for you, be prepared with several smart snacking solutions. Generally, snacks should be about 100–200 calories and low in saturated fat (definitely not more than 3 grams per serving, but the lower the better). The appropriate amount of carbohydrate in your snack depends on your blood glucose, activity level, and your meal plan. To learn how a particular snack affects your blood glucose, measure your blood glucose right before you eat and about two hours later. See Week 7 for more discussion about snacks, and, as always, talk to a registered dietitian to get a meal plan individualized for you.

SNACK OPTIONS

If you battle hunger between meals, choose a snack that combines protein and fiber. These two nutrients work together to keep you satisfied until mealtime. Below are a few good choices. You'll find more suggestions in the sample meal plans in the Appendix (page 183).

- Half sandwich (peanut butter, almond butter, tuna, or chicken on whole-grain, high-fiber bread)
- Hummus with bell peppers, carrots, cauliflower, or whole-wheat pita bread
- Low-fat or nonfat Greek yogurt and fruit (Greek yogurt is higher in protein than traditional yogurt, but both kinds are fine)
- Reduced-fat cheese or cottage cheese and raw veggies

BEAT HUNGER WITHOUT THE CARBS

Here are a few hunger-stopping options with limited carbohydrate for those times when your blood glucose is elevated or at the upper limit of your target range.

- ✦ Nuts: Choose any variety you like, but stick to one serving (¼ cup or 1 ounce). Pistachios are especially nice because the shells make the snack last longer, and each pistachio has only 3 or 4 calories.
- ✦ Reduced-fat cheese
- ✦ Hard-boiled egg
- ✦ Lettuce wrap: Place an ounce of turkey with shredded carrots and cucumber onto a romaine lettuce leaf, and wrap it up.
- ✦ Portobello "pizza:" Clean a Portobello mushroom and scrape the gills from the inside. Bake at 350°F for about 15 minutes, until soft. Remove the mushroom from the oven and fill the cavity with jarred spaghetti sauce, a sprinkling of shredded part-skim mozzarella cheese, and dried or fresh herbs of your choice. Add some chopped bell peppers, plum tomatoes, or other vegetables if you'd like. Broil for 1–2 minutes until the cheese is melted and a bit browned.
- ✦ Sliced tomato and other nonstarchy vegetables.

If heading straight for the refrigerator at the end of the day is your routine, you could undo all of the calorie savings from earlier in the day. A handful of this and a handful of that add up quickly. If you often eat as soon as you get home because you're over-hungry, a snack while at work or on the way home will help. Try one of the snacks on the previous page or have a piece of fruit or a few cups of popcorn. While you're preparing dinner or waiting for it to be ready, snack on salad vegetables. If you simply eat out of habit, change up your routine so the kitchen isn't your first stop. Enter the house through a different door and bypass the kitchen completely. Spend a few minutes relaxing, meditating, practicing yoga, or doing some other exercise before preparing meals or doing chores around your house.

CONQUER CRAVINGS

A craving is simply a strong desire, but sometimes that strong desire is so strong that it seems impossible to control. Some people more easily ignore cravings than others. While you may have had little success controlling food cravings previously, there are strategies that help.

Give Yourself Permission to Eat It

This is difficult for many dieters. So many people have the notion that weight loss and blood glucose control require giving up our favorite things. Really, though, it's about making choices and tradeoffs. Remember that you can have whatever you want, but you cannot have everything you want whenever you want it (or as much as you might want). Don't label the food as bad. Rather, eat a small bit of the food, savor every bite, thoroughly enjoy it, and remind yourself that yes, you can have it again another time. Once you really understand that it's okay to eat it and that you can have it again, the overwhelming desire to eat a lot disappears. In her book, *Eating Thin for Life*, Anne Fletcher, MS, RD, shares the dieting and maintenance strategies of 208 successful weight maintainers. These individuals have lost an average of 64 pounds and have kept it off for more than 10 years. The most frequent strategy for handling cravings? Having just a little.

Visualize Other Things

Australian researchers found that visualizing the appearance of a rainbow or other common sight curbs cravings. The theory is that cravings are strongest when you have a mental picture of the desired food, so replacing the mental image of the food with another image tames the cravings. When you're imagining a rainbow, for example, you're using up the brainpower that's needed to maintain cravings for pizza or chocolate. It may take a few attempts to get the hang of it, but it's something that you can try anywhere and anytime.

Chew on It

If you have a hankering for a snack, especially something sweet, reach for a stick of sugar-free gum instead of hitting the vending machine or raiding the pantry. A research study showed that when men and women chewed sugar-free gum for 15 minutes per hour in the afternoon, they reported less hunger, decreased cravings for sweets, and feeling more energetic than when they did not chew gum after lunch.

Find Balance

Take some "me" time. You deserve it. Get enough sleep, relax, and make time for fun to safeguard against those feelings of deprivation that often spark cravings.

MORE FROM LISA M.

"I think it's okay to go off the plan once in a while. It's very difficult to give up the once-loved foods we were used to eating before we were taught how to eat properly. I think every once in a while it's okay to treat yourself. It will keep you from giving up."

DISTRACT YOURSELF

You may be tempted to eat for reasons other than hunger and cravings. If you soothe a bad mood with food or find yourself grabbing something to eat because you have nothing better to do, it's time to distract yourself. Use these ideas to make a Distraction Kit. Keep your kit handy, just like you do with your Motivation Kit, so you can use it or add to it often and with ease. Look at the box on the next page for a few things you can include in your Distraction Kit.

OUTFITTING YOUR DISTRACTION KIT

- Exercise DVDs
- Exercise bands
- List of chores you never seem to get to, such as cleaning off your desk or workbench, organizing your drawer of kitchen utensils, and vacuuming the dust behind the furniture and window treatments.
- List of fun things you haven't made time for, such as learning to bead jewelry, organizing photos of your kids, figuring out how to use the apps you downloaded.
- Nail polish
- Deck of cards
- Notepaper and pens, blank greeting cards
- Puzzle book
- Joke book
- Magazines and catalogs
- Fancy bath oils or soaps

WEEK 12 ACTION STEPS

Continue your current goals or rewrite them if necessary. Additionally, select from the following goals or steps, modify them, or create your own. Choose goals from the previous weeks if applicable. This week I will:

☐ Continue the following goals: _____

_____

_____

☐ Eat snacks at planned times and only while hungry.

☐ Keep a list of acceptable snacks on the refrigerator door and keep the right foods handy.

☐ Carry sugar-free gum to work.

☐ Practice visualizing a rainbow or a favorite place to control my cravings.

☐ Allow myself a small bit of dessert at an appropriate time.

☐ Start my Distraction Kit.

☐ Buy nail polish, exercise bands, or _____.

☐ Other: _____

Week
13

Frequently dieters stick to what they think is a "safe routine," including eating the same meals they know fill them up and performing the same exercises they know how to do. The problem with keeping things the same is boredom and growing discontent—and that often leads to giving up. Boredom often hits around three months of following the same routine. That's why here, at Week 13, we look at ways to shake things up a bit. Being creative with meal replacements gives you more options at lunch and other times, and eating mindfully will bring more pleasure to your meals. Exercising in different places and trying new activities will keep your fitness plan fresh, too.

HAVE MEAL REPLACEMENTS HANDY

Mother Nature never dreamed of a meal in a can, but meal replacement bars and shakes may fill your need for a quick bite in our go, go, go, fast-paced society. Research studies show that dieters who use one or two meal replacements daily lose more weight than dieters following traditional weight-loss meal plans. Before you stock up on bars and cans, though, think carefully about the pros and cons of meal-replacement diets.

The Upside

The structure of using meal replacements makes sticking to a diet plan easier because you have fewer choices with which to struggle. You also get to eat as soon as you're hungry because there's no need to order or prepare food. There are no calories to count or portions to measure. You will still need to be aware of the carbohydrate content and the effects various meal replacements have on your blood glucose, however.

The Downside

It's not possible to get the same nutrition in a single packaged meal that you can get from a well-balanced home-prepared meal. Even those with ample protein, fiber, vitamins, and minerals still lack the disease-fighting phytochemicals Mother Nature so generously put into our fruits, vegetables, legumes, nuts, and grains. (Phytochemicals are compounds in plants that give the plant color, flavor, and aroma. There are thousands of them, and they work together to protect us from cancer, heart disease, age-related eye disease, and other illnesses.)

Meal replacements get boring. The same lack of choices that makes it easy to stick with the plan can eventually cause the diet doldrums and will have you seeking variety. If meal replacements keep you from eating with family and friends, the diet also becomes socially isolating.

Don't Skip...Replace

Meal replacements make ideal emergency meals. Keep a couple at home, at work, and even in your car to provide you with some nourishment when you might otherwise feel forced to skip a meal. Think beyond shakes and bars. Pick up a couple low-calorie frozen or shelf-stable meals that require no more preparation than microwaving. Use these guidelines for picking a meal replacement of any kind.

- 250–400 calories (for weight loss)
- at least 10 grams of protein
- at least 3 grams of fiber
- less than 3 grams of saturated fat
- less than 600 mg sodium for a frozen or shelf-stable meal and less than 300 mg sodium for bars and shakes
- at least 30% DV for most vitamins and minerals if you plan to use meal replacements regularly
- the carbohydrate content must match your individual needs and blood glucose goals
- add a piece of fruit to bulk up the meal and boost nutrients if you can make room for the extra carbohydrate
- add a salad to a small shelf-stable or frozen meal

PRACTICE EATING MINDFULLY

If you are fully aware of your food and how eating makes you feel, then you will enjoy your meal more and will likely become satisfied with less food. Paying such careful attention isn't as easy as it might seem, however. It requires that you take time to notice many aspects of your food and your body. It might also take superhuman strength to ignore the constant stream of noise and information we are all bombarded with nearly every minute of the day. (Think dogs, kids, Internet, email, smartphones!)

Try this: put two small, identical pieces of wrapped chocolate in front of you. Unwrap one, quickly toss it in your mouth, and eat it like you're in a race. Then open the second piece of chocolate, sniff it, turn it around in your fingers, look at its shape and texture, put it in your mouth and swirl it around with your tongue, slowly bite into it, notice its texture again, and savor it. Once the second piece of candy is gone, think about the experience and the pleasure the chocolate gave you compared with the experience of the first piece.

This candy experiment shows you that focusing on your food increases pleasure. Food is supposed to nourish our bodies, but it's also supposed to be pleasurable.

Mindful eating involves the following:

✦ Making choices about beginning and ending a meal based on awareness of the body's hunger and fullness cues. (Review the Hunger Ruler in Week 8 if necessary.)
✦ Choosing food that is enjoyable and nourishing.
✦ Eating without judging. Being aware of likes, dislikes, and neutral feelings without labeling the food or the experience as good or bad.
✦ Using senses other than taste to appreciate your food.

Try eating mindfully often. Give your food as much attention as you can. The more you practice eating mindfully, the easier it becomes.

FOR MORE INFORMATION

▮ The Center for Mindful Eating: www.tcme.org
▮ *Mindful Eating: A Guide to Rediscovering a Healthy and Joyful Relationship with Food* by Jan Chozen Bays, MD (Shambhala Publications, Inc., 2009)
▮ *Intuitive Eating: A Revolutionary Program that Works* by Evelyn Tribole, MS, RD, and Elyse Resch, MS, RD, FA, DA (St. Martin's Griffin, 2003)

REEVALUATE YOUR EXERCISE ROUTINE

You're approaching four months into your plan. If your exercise routine has become too boring, it's time to mix it up a bit. Why? After a while, your body adapts to doing the same exercises the same way and you benefit less from the time you put into it. And, since you're doing the same movements over and over, you're more likely to get injured. Finally, without varying your routine, you risk getting bored and quitting.

Shake up a stale exercise routine with any of these suggestions.

✦ Add intervals to your usual routine. If you walk, jog, or use any aerobic exercise machines, like the bike or rower, add several seconds to a few minutes of faster, higher-intensity exercise. Start out at your usual pace. After several minutes, sprint for one minute or some other comfortable amount of time. Return to your easier pace for several minutes and then sprint for another minute. Do several cycles of this. For example, if you usually exercise at a moderate intensity level of 12–14 on the Borg Rate of Perceived Exertion (RPE) Scale (see Week 3 for a refresher on RPE), throw in a few intervals at level 15 or 16 for several seconds to a minute at a time. As you get into better shape, increase the frequency and length of your intervals. You'll like the results.

✦ Vary your exercise type. If you always walk, hop on the bike once or twice per week. If you always use the treadmill, take a walk outside.

✦ Sign up for a fitness challenge, such as a charity 5K walk or run.

✦ Join a fitness class.

✦ Find a fitness buddy who can encourage you to try new things.

✦ Treat yourself to a new gadget, such as a heart rate monitor, a stability ball, a Zumba Fitness exercise DVD, elastic exercise bands, or a new program for your gaming system.

✦ Seek help from a personal trainer.

HOW TO PICK A PERSONAL TRAINER

A personal trainer should customize your workouts for you, teach you to work out safely, challenge you to do better, and provide motivation.

✦ Choose a trainer who has been certified by a nationally recognized and accredited certifying organization, such as the American College of Sports Medicine (ACSM), American Council on Exercise (ACE), Cooper Institute, National Academy of Sports Medicine (NASM), National Council on Strength and Fitness (NCSF), National Exercise

Trainers Association (NETA), National Federation of Professional Trainers (NFPT), or National Strength and Conditioning Association (NSCA). There are many, many certifications, and some require very little training. Be certain to take time to learn about your trainer's credentials.

- ✦ Find out if the trainer is trained to perform CPR.
- ✦ Ask about education. Many trainers have college degrees in exercise science and many do not.
- ✦ Discuss your health and any complications with the trainer. Be certain to hire someone with experience working with people similar to you.
- ✦ Ask for references, and check them.
- ✦ Chat with the trainer in person or on the phone to be sure you are a good fit for each other.
- ✦ Learn about the trainer's cancellation policy and how billing is handled.
- ✦ Be certain your trainer carries liability insurance.
- ✦ Take nutrition advice only if your personal trainer is also a registered dietitian. Additionally, your trainer should not offer medical advice.

HOW TO PICK A GYM

A gym can be a place where you work out regularly or just once or twice a week between other activities. For example, you may prefer to get your aerobic activity by playing tennis and walking around your neighborhood, but hit the gym for a dance class or to lift weights. Ask yourself the following questions when selecting a gym.

- ✦ Is it conveniently located and are the hours of operation convenient? Does it provide childcare?
- ✦ Is it too crowded during the hours you want to be there? Be certain to visit during those same hours.
- ✦ Are the facilities and equipment clean and in working order?
- ✦ Is the staff trained?
- ✦ Is there an AED (automated external defibrillator) should someone on site have a heart attack?
- ✦ Does it offer the fitness classes and programs you want? Is there enough variety to keep your interest?
- ✦ Are the contract and cost agreeable to you? Can you have a one-week free pass to try out the gym? Can you put your membership on hold if you are injured or have lengthy travel?

MORE FROM HENRY S.

❝ I wanted to avoid—and hopefully reverse—the loss of muscle mass that occurs with weight loss and aging. I know that walking isn't enough to take care of that. Given my age, lack of fitness, diabetic neuropathy, arthritis, occasional dizzy spells, and lack of confidence, I got a recommendation for a personal trainer skilled at working with individuals similar to me. I work with her about once a week, and I do some of the exercises on my own, too. I can clearly do more work and with less soreness since I started with her a little more than two months ago. As my confidence continues to grow, I'll do more and more work on my own and see her less frequently. ❞

WEEK 13 ACTION STEPS

Continue your current goals or rewrite them if necessary. Additionally, select from the following goals or steps, modify them, or create your own. Choose goals from the previous weeks if applicable. This week I will:

☐ Continue the following goals: _____ _____

_____ _____

_____

☐ Buy a few meal replacements to have on hand for super busy days.

☐ Practice eating mindfully at least once each day.

☐ Sign up for an exercise class or check out a new exercise DVD at the library.

☐ Add intervals to my morning walk at least once.

☐ Ask friends to recommend a personal trainer.

☐ Add to my Distraction Kit.

☐ Review my Motivation Kit.

☐ Try at least one new recipe.

☐ Check out the restaurant nutrition information before going out to dinner.

☐ Other: _____

Week 14

Continuing on last week's theme of fighting or preventing diet doldrums and boredom, this week we look at adding interest to both your food and your beverages. We also introduce the topic of binge eating.

MAKE WATER YOUR GO-TO DRINK

At least 50% of a healthy adult's body weight is fluid. What could be better than life-sustaining water to quench your thirst, hydrate your body, and flush away toxins? Although all beverages provide fluids, water doesn't contain coloring, sugars, artificial sweeteners, and calories. If you're not a fan of water, now is a good time to become one. Sometimes an inexpensive water filter pitcher or faucet attachment is good enough to brighten the taste of water. If you want something a little more flavorful, experiment with these flavor enhancers.

- ✦ Cucumber slices. Add them to a pitcher of water and refrigerate overnight.
- ✦ Cucumber and orange slices.
- ✦ Fresh mint.
- ✦ Cucumber, lemon, mint, and rosemary.
- ✦ Lemon or orange slices or both.
- ✦ Squeeze of fresh citrus or all-natural citrus flavor like True Lemon.
- ✦ Unsweetened iced or freshly brewed tea, plain or with any of the above flavorings.
- ✦ Unflavored seltzer water mixed with a splash of cranberry, pomegranate, cherry, or grape juice. (This is no longer calorie or carb-free, so account for the juice in your meal plan.)

In theory, for every 3,500 calories you save, you'll lose one pound. If you drink a lot of caloric beverages, you may not realize how quickly they add up. A single can of soda will cost you about 150 calories, as will 8–12 ounces of fruit juice. Replace just one of these drinks each day, and you'll save the amount of calories in a pound of body fat in just three to four weeks. Replace two drinks with water daily and you save those same calories in half the time. This is a great example of how making small changes adds up to big results over time.

JAZZ UP YOUR MEALS

Water isn't the only thing that might get boring. A lot of people don't think nutritious and delicious go together or think they have to have gourmet cooking skills to bake a flavorful chicken breast. Not true. What you need is a little creativity, some extra time to experiment, a good cookbook or website, and the ability to shrug off things that don't work out. Here are a few ideas to jazz up a simple meal.

- ✦ Before baking a boneless, skinless chicken breast, coat it with crumbs of one kind or another to trap in the moisture and to add flavor. You can make the crumbs stick by first dipping the chicken into egg, egg white, egg substitute, or a bit of milk. You can even brush the chicken first with reduced-fat ranch or peppercorn dressing for a kick of flavor.
  - ▮ Italian-seasoned bread crumbs with or without a little Parmesan cheese
  - ▮ Cornflake crumbs with orange zest, cinnamon, and brown sugar
  - ▮ Seasoned quick-cooking oats
- ✦ Mix just a spoonful of pesto sauce into cooked grains like rice or quinoa and into vegetable and chicken soups.
- ✦ Sprinkle a small amount of nuts or pungent cheese into salads, vegetables, and grains.
- ✦ Cook fruit instead of eating it raw.
- ✦ Experiment with flavored vinegars. Try a splash on a green salad, steamed vegetables, potato salad, and soups and stews.
- ✦ Brighten grilled or baked fish and chicken with a salsa of fruit and herbs.
- ✦ Soak dried mushrooms in hot water for about 15 minutes or until they become soft. Add them to stews, soups, vegetable medleys, and more. Use the strained soaking liquid in soups and stews and to enhance flavors when braising meats.

+ Add interest with variety. For example, if making a tomato-based dish, use a combination of canned, fresh, and sun-dried tomatoes.

JAZZY RECIPES

These recipes in the Appendix will help you add pizzazz to your everyday cooking. They use common ingredients in not-so-common ways.

- Crispy Chicken Dijon
- Lemony Asparagus Spear Salad
- Salmon Fillets with Pineapple Salsa
- Chunky Greek-Style Salad with Tuna
- Grilled Fresh Mission Figs

IDENTIFY BINGE EATING

Everyone occasionally stuffs himself or herself, but if it's more than an occasional binge and if it's accompanied with a terrible out-of-control feeling, you may need someone to help you find balance and take charge of your eating. About 3% of adults in the U.S. have a binge eating disorder. Many people with this problem are reluctant to seek help because they're too embarrassed, they fear ridicule, or because they don't know that things can be better. If you see yourself in the following description on more than a rare occasion, gather your courage and speak to your physician about a referral to a qualified mental health professional. The results can change your life.

+ Eating large amounts of food in a short period of time, even when you're full
+ Eating secretly
+ Frequently eating until uncomfortably full
+ Feeling out of control while eating and guilty or disgusted with yourself after eating

WEEK 14 ACTION STEPS

Continue your current goals or rewrite them if necessary. Additionally, select from the following goals or steps, modify them, or create your own. Choose goals from the previous weeks if applicable. This week I will:

☐ Continue the following goals: _____

_____

_____

☐ Buy a water filter.

☐ Keep a pitcher of ice-cold flavored water available.

☐ Buy and use exotic vinegar or pesto sauce.

☐ Grill fruit.

☐ Sign up for a healthy cooking class at the community center.

☐ Speak to my physician about binge eating.

☐ Recommit to keeping a food record.

☐ Make a walking date instead of a lunch date.

☐ Other: _____

Week 15

Planning has helped you be successful these last 14 weeks. You've planned for breakfasts, parties, grocery shopping, exercise, and more. Now we look at back-up plans.

MAKE PLAN B

The best plans still fail now and then. And the best planners have a back-up plan for those days when nothing seems to go right. Your child is sick, your boss moved up your deadline, traffic is a mess, or your bagged lunch is still sitting on the kitchen counter. Even though it doesn't always seem like it, there's usually a way to get a healthful meal no matter what throws a wrench into your plan. By anticipating some problems and their solutions, you'll be able to stay on track. Here are some suggestions to get you through interruptions to your schedule. Your own ideas are probably better, so brainstorm some solutions to common problems. Make a written list and keep it where you'll see it when you need it.

6 Quick-and-Easy Dinners to Throw Together

Be sure to keep your pantry and freezer stocked with ready-to-eat staples. These aren't gourmet meals, but they're tasty, nutritious, and oh so fast.

1. Toasted cheese sandwich (whole-wheat bread and reduced-fat cheese); reduced-sodium canned vegetable soup; fresh, frozen, or canned fruit.
2. Reduced-sodium black bean or lentil soup, bagged salad, sliced apple, or other fruit.

3. Whole-grain pasta, jarred pasta sauce, any of the following: rinsed canned cannellini beans, canned clams, or frozen soy crumbles. Toss in any leftover or frozen vegetables you have on hand.
4. Frozen stir-fry vegetables mixed with instant brown rice and cooked shrimp or chicken from your freezer.
5. Tuna salad on bagged lettuce; whole-grain crackers; fresh, frozen, or canned fruit.
6. Fat-free refried beans, no-salt-added canned tomatoes (drained), canned chile peppers, and reduced-fat cheddar cheese mixed together in a baking dish and heated in the oven or microwave. Serve with soft corn or whole-wheat tortillas and jarred salsa.

2 Dinners to Grab on the Way Home

Instead of stopping at the fast food restaurant when you're running late, feeling tired, and hungry for dinner, dash into your local supermarket.

1. Rotisserie chicken, small baking potatoes to microwave, frozen green nonstarchy vegetables.
2. Steamed shrimp (order this at the fish counter when you first arrive; it usually takes about 5 minutes), bagged coleslaw, and light dressing to mix at home, pre-cut fruit.

7 Emergency Foods to Stash at Work or in the Car

Don't you just hate that feeling of being hungry but you've got nothing to eat? If you need a snack while working late, you're stuck in traffic, or if you forgot to bring your lunch to work, one of these will satisfy.

1. Frozen or shelf-stable meal: see Week 13 for guidelines on picking one.
2. Larabars: made of fruit and nuts. Buy the minis to keep the calories at 100 or less and the carbohydrates between 10 and 14 grams.
3. Pistachios: You can eat 25–30 for about 100 calories. The shells will slow you down, too, making your snack last longer and more satisfying.
4. Shelled nuts in ⅛- or ¼-cup servings: pre-measure nuts and store them in small baggies or use an old mint tin.
5. Kashi granola bar or other brand made of whole grains.
6. Individual packets of natural peanut butter or almond butter and whole-wheat crackers or pretzels.

7. Dash by the grocery store to pick up a piece of fruit or a cup of low-fat yogurt. Ask at the deli counter for a plastic spoon for the yogurt.

Fast Food and Take Out

This section is entirely up to you. To be in control when plan A falls apart, know what you'll order before the time comes. Write the names of each of your favorite fast-food and take-out restaurants on the top of an index card. Under the restaurant name, write one or more full meals you can order. This way you won't have to do any calorie or carbohydrate math or be tempted by something unhealthful when hunger strikes. Keep one index card for every restaurant you frequent, and keep those cards near the phone, in the car, or wherever you will need them for reference. You might even need more than one set, so you can find them in all the places you could need them.

WEEK 15 ACTION STEPS

Continue your current goals or rewrite them if necessary. Additionally, select from the following goals or steps, modify them, or create your own. Choose goals from the previous weeks if applicable. This week I will:

☐ Continue the following goals: _____

_____

_____

☐ Stock up on pantry staples for fast, healthful meals.

☐ Create a list of meals to put together quickly. Explain it to my family members, so they can get dinner ready when I'm late getting home.

☐ Buy healthful snacks to keep in the car and at work. Store them where I don't see them, but can get them when I need them.

☐ Make a list of the best choices for the five take-out restaurants I call most often. Keep that list in my smartphone and at home where my family can use it.

☐ Try out another exercise DVD from the library.

☐ Other: _____

Week 16

After nearly four months, it's a good time to reflect on your diet and fine-tune your weight-loss plan to include the most nutritious foods with a variety of disease fighters. Additionally, if you are still struggling with some very important goals, asking for help may make all the difference.

WHAT'S ON YOUR PLATE?

It's easy to forget about balance and focus only on carbohydrates when you are struggling to control blood glucose, or focus only on calories when trying to lose weight, or just on sodium when thinking about blood pressure. Unfortunately, none of us has the luxury of giving all of our attention to such a narrow slice of our diet. The expression "a chain is only as strong as its weakest link" is applicable to diet. Eating lots of vegetables and few desserts is a good thing, but it doesn't make up for eating large amounts of refined grains and fatty meats, for example. Examine your diet with this quiz to find your weak links.

1. Do you eat fish that is not fried at least twice weekly?
   ____yes   ____no

2. Do you eat at least 2 cups of beans or lentils weekly?
   ____yes   ____no

3. Do you eat at least 1 cup of fruit each day?
   ____yes   ____no

4. Do you eat at least 2 cups of vegetables each day?
   ____yes   ____no

5. Do you eat dark green vegetables at least 4 times each week?
____yes ____no

6. Do you eat red or orange vegetables most days of the week?
____yes ____no

7. Do you limit fried foods to no more than one small serving each week?
____yes ____no

8. When you eat poultry, do you remove the skin?
____yes ____no

9. When you eat beef, do you choose only lean cuts and trim away the visible fat?
____yes ____no

10. When using ground meat (even for poultry), do you use only 90% lean or a higher number?
____yes ____no

11. Most of the time, do you use soft or liquid fats (tub margarine and oil) instead of hard fats (butter, stick margarine, lard, bacon grease, vegetable shortening) for cooking, seasoning, and spreading?
____yes ____no

12. Do you avoid sugary drinks?
____yes ____no

13. Do you limit processed foods with added sugars (such as a granola bar) to no more than one very small serving daily?
____yes ____no

14. Do you limit added sugars (honey, molasses, agave nectar, brown sugar, syrup, etc.) to no more than 1 tablespoon daily?
____yes ____no

15. Do you eat blue/purple fruits and vegetables at least three times weekly?
____yes ____no

16. Do you eat white/brown fruits and vegetables at least three times weekly?
____yes ____no

17. Do you eat yellow/orange fruits and vegetables at least three times weekly?
____yes ____no

18. Do you eat at least three servings of whole grains every day?
____yes ____no

19. Do you limit refined grains to no more than two servings each day?
____yes ____no

20. Do you eat nuts, seeds, and nut butters at least three times per week but limit each occasion to just 1 ounce?
____yes ____no

21. Do you limit alcohol to one drink per day if you are female and to two drinks per day if you are male (saving up to drink extra on some days is NOT acceptable)?
____yes ____no

22. Do you use reduced-sodium products at home whenever possible?
____yes ____no

23. Do you enjoy your food most of the time?
____yes ____no

24. Do you eat only the amount of food to satisfy your hunger most of the time?
____yes ____no

This is not a perfect quiz, but it will help you identify areas that need attention. For every question that you answered no, think about improvements you're willing to make. Write down your SMART goals and start making better choices today.

MORE FROM MICHAEL B.

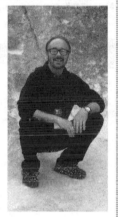

❝ I've lost weight before, but I didn't keep it off. My problem started when I gave up running because my knees were hurting. My schedule got crazy, and I started eating all the wrong kinds of convenience foods. I gained more and more weight back. This time it's different in two ways. First, losing weight is all about my life and my health. Before it was cosmetic. Second, this time I rely on healthful, whole foods instead of going without eating. Before, I went to bed hungry and had to fight not to eat a lot. This time I'm eating better foods, and it controls my hunger. I'm about 80% vegetarian. Sometimes I eat chicken, turkey, or fish. I can get lots of protein from beans and other veggies. I love that I did this without a special diet plan. I lost weight by simply eating healthy foods. My blood glucose is controlled. I love that. And I feel better. I usually got sick at least once in the fall and again in the spring. I have not been sick in over a year. That's cool! ❞

FOR MORE INFORMATION

A registered dietitian is the perfect person to help you tweak your diet. You can ask your physician for a referral or find a dietitian in your area by visiting the Academy of Nutrition and Dietetics website (*www.eatright.org*). Click on Find a Dietitian and enter your zip code. Fortunately, insurance providers frequently cover dietitian appointments for people with diabetes. Call your insurance company to find out about your coverage. You can also track your food intake at the American Diabetes Association's MyFoodAdvisor™ (*www.diabetes.org*).

ASK FOR HELP

There are few successes in life that one achieves alone. Healthful eating, weight loss, and blood glucose control are not exceptions. Getting help and support from others is critical to achieving success with these goals, just as it is with raising children, learning to drive, woodworking, mastering algebra, and most other skills and goals. Sometimes it seems like asking for support is a weakness, but it's not. It's smart to get the help you need. By taking care of you, you're better able to take care of others. And by investing in yourself today, you'll be in better shape in your later years. Your health care costs will be less and your ability to work and enjoy life will be greater.

To get the help you need, ask in a way to make yourself understood.

+ **Be direct.** Often it's tempting to hint, but there are two problems with this. First, your family or friends may not catch your hint and, therefore, not help you appropriately. Second, they may fully understand what you want, but resent that you're not being honest or clear. If you need someone else to do some chores to allow you time to exercise, just ask in a straightforward way. "Can you clean the supper dishes, so I can take a walk in the evenings?" This is much nicer and more effective than hinting: "If I just didn't have so much to do in the evenings, I could finally get some exercise."

+ **Be specific about what and why.** "Stop hassling me about what I eat," could mean a lot of things. "I'd like it if you wouldn't comment on my food choices because I think you don't understand my meal plan," says everything the other person needs to know.

- **Educate your family and friends.** A lot of people want to help, but don't know how. By teaching them about diabetes and your meal plan and by sharing how you feel about diabetes and trying to lose weight, they'll understand more about what you need to be successful.
- **Pass out the Diabetes Etiquette card.** When all else fails, download and hand out this brilliant card published by the Behavioral Diabetes Institute (www.behavioraldiabetesinstitute.org). It offers 10 Dos and Don'ts for family and friends of people with diabetes. Many are applicable to your weight-loss efforts, too.

VINCENT S'S STORY

" My biggest supporter and manager is my wife, Patricia. I used to eat a lot of cakes, cookies, and chocolate. Now we keep it out of the house, even though Patricia doesn't need to avoid it like I do. We've talked about how I'm supposed to eat, so she makes sure that half my dinner plate is filled with vegetables. It would be very hard to do this without all of Patricia's support. "

Finding a Diabetes Support Group

Sometimes the best support is not from family and close friends. Rather, it's from people who struggle with the same issues as you. A diabetes support group is just the place to find such people. There will be people there who understand the challenges of managing a diet for both diabetes and weight control. They'll know what it's like to have friends who say the wrong thing when they are trying to say the right thing. And they will know what diet and diabetes burnout feel like. To find a local support group, visit the American Diabetes Association's *In My Community* (www.diabetes.org/in-my-community). You should also ask your physician or your diabetes educator for recommendations, and make calls to the local hospitals. If you're fortunate to have several in your area, visit a few to find the group that feels the most comfortable. Ask about online support groups and communities, too, but use caution. Some that look legitimate are merely unscrupulous people looking to sell you expensive supplements or diet plans. If you have any doubts about the trustworthiness of an online group or program, ask a health professional to help you evaluate it.

WEEK 16 ACTION STEPS

Continue your current goals or rewrite them if necessary.
Additionally, select from the following goals or steps,
modify them, or create your own. Choose goals from the previous
weeks if applicable. This week I will:

☐ Continue the following goals: _____

_____

_____

☐ Examine my food record for dietary weaknesses.

☐ Eat healthfully prepared fish at least twice.

☐ Find a new recipe for beans.

☐ Call around for a diabetes support group.

☐ Ask my spouse to take a walk with me after dinner at least once.

☐ Other: _____

Part 2

FOCUSING ON THE LONG TERM

Congratulations! You have practiced a lot of skills and tried out new strategies in the last 16 weeks. Good for you! Certainly some weeks were harder than others, and some skills have been harder to master than others. These skills will carry you far in your quest for a healthy, fun-filled life. So keep at it, consistency is key.

To keep you focused long term, this book's plan spans a full year. Here we switch to a month-by-month schedule and introduce additional skills you'll need to make your plan work for the long haul. In these next chapters, we'll talk about reducing sodium, shopping on a budget, and more.

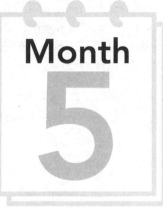

Month 5

This month we expand on last week's goal of fine-tuning your food choices. We reinforce eating a variety of foods to keep you healthy and to make your diet program livable for the long term. Stress management skills are also necessary for your ongoing success, so we take a look at those, too.

FOR THE LONG HAUL: STAY OUT OF A FOOD RUT

The same breakfast day after day followed by the same lunch gets tiresome. Even if you prefer it that way because it's easy, fast, and comfortable, it breaks the first rule of good nutrition: *Eat a variety of foods.* No single food provides all the nutrients you need for good health. In fact, it takes a shopping cart of different foods to even come close. Vitamins, minerals, protein, fiber, and antioxidants are just the tip of the iceberg.

Scientists have discovered thousands of phytochemicals, compounds in plants that help prevent disease, and they discover new, important phytochemicals all the time. "Phytochemical" literally means "plant chemical." The term describes the compounds in fruits, vegetables, nuts, beans, and grains that give the plant color, aroma, and flavor and protect the plant from microbial infestation and other diseases. In the diet, phytochemicals work together and with other nutrients to fend off heart disease, age-related eye disease, cancer, and more. Among their many functions, phytochemicals might prevent DNA damage, boost the immune system, and help relax blood vessels. The only way to get enough of these health-boosting phytochemicals is to eat a variety of plant foods.

Break out of a food rut by starting a supper club among friends, picking a new food each week at the supermarket, shopping in an ethnic market or buying an ethnic cookbook, taking a cooking class, eating fruits and vegetables from each color palette every day, and randomly opening a healthy cookbook to find your next new recipe.

10 FOODS FOR EVERY GROCERY LIST

This is not even close to a full list of recommended foods. It's simply meant to help you think past your usual list.

Barley: This grain is rich in beta-glucan, a fiber that's good for your cholesterol and glucose levels. Toss it in soups and stews, substitute it for pasta in salads, and for rice in side dishes.

Edamame Beans: Keep these high-fiber, high-protein beans in your freezer for a quick, easy snack or lunch. Simply boil the beans, still in their pods, for about five minutes. Sprinkle lightly with salt, if desired.

Beets: Get a serving of blue/purple produce with fully cooked, ready-to-eat packaged beets. Find them in the cold section of your grocer's produce department or buy fresh beets and roast them with a little olive oil.

Greek Yogurt: Thicker than regular yogurt, Greek yogurt is a creamy, delicious source of protein and other nutrients. It's perfect for desserts, smoothies, and cream sauces, and as a replacement for sour cream.

Lentils: Unlike other dried legumes, lentils don't need to be pre-soaked. They're loaded with potassium, fiber, and a host of other nutrients. Make soups, salads, and even mix lentils with ground meat in meatloaf and burgers.

Mango: Every fruit belongs on this list, but mango is here because it's frequently a mystery to people and is more versatile than you probably realize. Choose slightly firm, sweet-smelling mangoes with a variety of colors on the skin. Enjoy mango fresh by itself or with other fruit, purée it in smoothies, add diced mango to rice, and swap out some or all of the tomato for mango in your favorite salsa recipe.

Nut Butters: Choose peanut butter, almond butter, or any other kind of nut butter. They all contain good-for-you fats. Buy one variety this month and a different kind next month. Think beyond the sandwich; enjoy nut butters spread on apple slices and mixed into Asian-inspired recipes.

Pistachios and Other Nuts: Pistachios are called the "skinny nut" because they're only 3–4 calories each and because the shells help you with portion control. Choose these and all the other nuts you love. Just use restraint because an ounce of nuts varies from about 160 to 200 calories.

Quinoa: Pronounced "keen-wah," this high-protein grain cooks up in about 15 minutes. Use it in place of rice or any starch. Served cold with veggies and a vinaigrette, quinoa is delicious as a main-dish salad.

Sardines: These tiny fish are a great source of omega-3 fatty acids. Buy a few cans when they're on sale because they'll stay fresh for a couple of years. Toss them onto a mixed salad or spread mashed sardines on crackers.

ADDRESS STRESS

Life is stressful, and having diabetes makes it even more stressful. For some, emotional stress may produce hormones that send blood glucose surging or increase food cravings. The best stress beater is preventing it in the first place, though that is much easier said than done. Stress prevention basics include the following:

+ Get plenty of sleep
+ Engage in regular exercise
+ Eat healthfully
+ Enjoy "me time" every day
+ Spend time with family and friends
+ Confide in someone
+ Set realistic goals
+ Ask for help when you're busier than usual
+ Do something that makes you chuckle: see a funny movie, read the comics, watch the little kids down the street play

BREATHING EXERCISES

Some people find stress relief in jogging, yoga, meditation, progressive muscle relaxation, and other ways. Breathing exercises work for many, and you can do them anywhere.

In a comfortable, relaxed position, inhale deeply through your nose and exhale through your mouth. Your abdomen should rise when you breathe in, but your chest should move very little. Imagine that each incoming breath brings energy, and try to visualize the energy traveling to each part of your body. As you exhale, picture your breath cleansing your body of all its stored tension.

MONTH 5 ACTION STEPS

Continue your current goals or rewrite them if necessary. Additionally, select from the following goals or steps, modify them, or create your own. Choose goals from the previous weeks if applicable. This month I will:

☐ Continue the following goals: _____

_____

_____

☐ Ask friends at work to join me in trying new lunch recipes.

☐ Prepare at least one new grain recipe and two new entrées.

☐ Buy produce in every color.

☐ Buy nuts in single-serve packages for snacks.

☐ Practice breathing exercises for stress management.

☐ Make a point to observe or do something funny every day.

☐ Other: _____

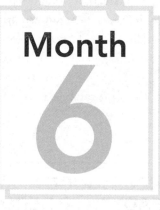

Month 6

Many dieters find that weight loss stalls after about six months, so here we address the dreaded plateau. But first, we give special attention to the types of fats in your foods—again to make your diet plan work for the long term. Pay attention to more tricky food labels!

FOR THE LONG HAUL: LIMIT SATURATED AND TRANS FATS

There's no need to drastically limit the amount of fat you eat. Fat enhances the taste and mouth-feel of your food, and it helps you absorb fat-soluble nutrients. Having a little bit of fat with your salad, for example, helps you absorb some of the nutrients in your greens and tomatoes.

The problem with fat is that it has a lot of calories—more than twice as many as in carbohydrate and protein, so watch your total fat intake to keep calories in check. The other problem is that two types of fats (saturated and trans fats) likely raise your risk of heart disease, cause unwanted inflammation linked to type 2 diabetes, and lead to a host of other health problems. These are the ones to avoid. According to the *Dietary Guidelines for Americans, 2010*, we consume too much saturated and trans fats. To trim your intake, indulge only occasionally in small amounts of pizza, full-fat cheese, and other full-fat dairy, baked goods, sausage, bacon, hot dogs, ribs, poultry skin, fatty meats, fried foods, butter, stick margarine, shortening, and other solid fats. In their place, enjoy moderate amounts of foods containing good-for-you fats like nuts and seeds, nut butters, vegetable oils, and avocado. At home, cook with canola, soybean, or olive oils instead of butter or lard. Use a low saturated-fat soft spread for toast. Slip a slice of avocado into your sandwich instead of cheese, and make a sandwich with almond butter or peanut butter instead of bologna. In restaurants, order a small baked potato instead of French fries. At the supermarket, check the Nutrition Facts panel for both saturated and trans fats. Additionally, look at the ingredients list to avoid groceries containing partially hydrogenated oils, a telltale sign that the product contains trans fats. Look at the two sample food labels on the following pages and see how simple it can be to identify these fats and the fat-providing ingredients.

CHEESY RICE
READY IN 90 SECONDS
Nutrition Facts

Serving Size 1 cup (230g)
Servings Per Container 2

Amount Per Serving

Calories 250	**Calories from Fat** 100

	% Daily Value*
Total Fat 11g	**17%**
Saturated Fat 3g	**15%**
Trans Fat 1g	
Cholesterol 35mg	**12%**
Sodium 325mg	**14%**
Total Carbohydrate 33g	**11%**
Dietary Fiber 0g	**0%**
Sugars 4g	
Protein 4g	

Calories per gram:
Fat 9 • Carbohydrate 4 • Protein 4

Ingredients: WATER, LONG GRAIN PARBOILED RICE, SOYBEAN OIL, SALT, PARTIALLY HYDROGENATED SOYBEAN OIL, PARMESAN, CHEDDAR, SWISS, ROMANO CHEESES, MODIFIED CORN STARCH, LACTIC ACID, WHEY, HYDROLYZED CORN PROTEIN, NONFAT MILK, TURMERIC (COLOR), NATURAL FLAVORS, SPICE, NIACIN, THIAMINE MONO-NITRATE, FOLIC ACID, RIBOFLAVIN, FERROUS SULFATE

The cheese is the likely source of most of the saturated fat, and the hydrogenated soybean oil provides the trans fat. If you ate just one cup of the prepared rice, you would have eaten 3 grams of saturated fat and 1 gram of trans fat. Some people will eat the entire package (2 servings), logging 6 grams of saturated fat and 2 grams of trans fat. Remember: always look at the serving size first because every other number relates to that amount of food.

DINNER ROLL
Nutrition Facts

Serving Size 1 roll (65g)
Servings Per Container 6

Amount Per Serving

Calories 180	**Calories from Fat** 45

% Daily Value*

Total Fat 5g	**8%**
Saturated Fat 2g	**10%**
Trans Fat 0g	
Cholesterol 0mg	**0%**
Sodium 380mg	**16%**
Total Carbohydrate 30g	**10%**
Dietary Fiber 1g	**4%**
Sugars 3g	
Protein 4g	

Calories per gram:
Fat 9   •   Carbohydrate 4   •   Protein 4

Ingredients: ENRICHED FLOUR (wheat flour, niacin, ferrous sulfate, thiamin mononitrate, riboflavin, folic acid), WATER, SOYBEAN OIL, SUGAR, PARTIALLY HYDROGENATED COTTENSEED OIL, LEAVENING (baking soda, glucono delta lactone), SALT, NATURAL and ARTIFICIAL FLAVOR, YEAST, XANTHAN GUM, AUTOLYZED YEAST EXTRACT

You might think that these rolls have no trans fat. Not so fast. Yes, the Nutrition Facts panel clearly says that one roll has 0 g of trans fat. Though *legally* accurate, this is not *technically* accurate. Manufacturers are allowed to claim that any food containing less than 0.5 grams of trans fat has 0 grams of trans fat. Therefore, even for foods that appear to be trans-fat free, read the ingredients list. In this case, you'll find partially hydrogenated cottonseed oil, a source of trans fats. All partially hydrogenated oils will provide at least a trace amount of trans fat.

If you eat a roll or two and perhaps a serving or two of a soft spread also made with partially hydrogenated oils and some packaged foods earlier in the day, all of those trace amounts can add up to more than your daily limit. Do your best to avoid everything with partially hydrogenated oils. Claims like "Low Fat" or "Trans Fat Free" on the packaging are enticing, but it's the Nutrition Facts panel and the ingredients list that give you the real information.

How Much Is Too Much?

Recommended Daily Limit	1,300 Calories	1,500 Calories	1,800 Calories	2,000 Calories
Saturated Fat	14 g	16 g	20 g	22 g
Trans Fat*	1 g	1 g	2 g	2 g

* A few foods contain naturally occurring trans fats, but since they also provide important nutrients, the *Guidelines* do not recommend eliminating them. This means it's even more important to strictly limit the "industrial" or "synthetic" trans fats produced when foods are fried or when manufacturers use partially hydrogenated oils.

SEEK OUT THE GOOD-FOR-YOU FATS

Don't forget to include sources of omega-3 fatty acids. There are two types of these health-boosting fats: those found in some fish and those found in some plants. Both types are linked to a healthy heart. Research suggests that the omega-3 fats in fish may also promote brain and eye development in infants and children, improve the cognitive function of the elderly, and lessen the symptoms of inflammatory diseases such as arthritis, asthma, and ulcerative colitis. Choose foods with omega-3 fats often, such as:

✦ Walnuts, ground flaxseed, tofu, soybeans, canola and soybean oils, bluefish, herring, lake trout, mackerel, salmon, sardines, tuna

Other good-for-you fats include the monounsaturated fats found in nuts, avocados, olive, soybean, and canola oils, and olives. Be very careful not to add these high-fat foods to your diet without eliminating other foods. You'll likely gain weight without replacing one food for another. A good swap is trading cheese for avocado or chips for nuts. Use them sparingly, however.

BUSTING THROUGH PLATEAUS

Most successful dieters hit the dreaded weight-loss plateau eventually. Frequently, it occurs after about six months of weight loss or when the individual has lost about 10% of his or her starting weight (about 20 pounds for someone starting at 200 pounds). As hugely frustrating as the plateau is, it's not the time to throw in the towel. A lot of people get so frustrated with the lack of weight loss that they just quit trying or they make radical diet changes, mistakenly believing that it's necessary to "shake up the body" to start losing again. Your body doesn't need shocking or shaking up. What has happened is the new, smaller you burns fewer calories than the old, larger you. If it feels that you have to cut back even more than before only to lose weight at a slower pace or not at all, you are correct. It seems like a dirty trick, but it's just the way the body works. Instead of letting this break your motivation, increase your focus to break through the plateau.

- **Go back to the basics.** When you first started this weight-loss plan, you probably took more care to keep records, measure your food, and plan ahead than you do now. Get back to those first behaviors. If your measuring cups are collecting dust, you might be surprised that your ½-cup serving of pasta has blossomed to ¾ cup.
- **Make a date with yourself.** Spend some quiet time reflecting on why you have worked so hard and why you want to continue your weight loss. Grab your Motivation Kit, and review your list of reasons to lose weight. Add more reasons as you think of them.
- **Visualize the result.** Spend a couple minutes each morning seeing yourself looking and feeling fabulous.
- **Make two or three food swaps every day.** For example, have an open-faced sandwich for lunch instead of your typical sandwich or trade in your 6-ounce juice glass for a 4-ounce glass. Or, consider having a piece of fruit instead of juice.
- **Start every lunch and dinner with nonstarchy vegetables.** Broccoli, zucchini, cabbage, tomatoes, and more are low in calories and can help take the edge off your appetite before you dig into the higher-calorie foods.
- **Watch your alcohol intake.** Not only does the alcohol have calories, but drinking might weaken your resolve to cut back on high-calorie food.
- **Rev up your workout.** If you aren't already lifting weights or performing some other type of resistance exercise, get started. Next, add intervals to your aerobic exercise routine. See Weeks 1, 3, 4, 6, 7, and 12 to review the information about exercise. Go on a workout tour by visiting a new class at a gym every day or every other day for a week.
- **Wear a pedometer.** If you haven't yet bought one or if you've pushed yours into the back of a drawer, clip on a pedometer and challenge

yourself to more and more steps each day. See Week 1 for information about selecting and wearing a pedometer.

✦ **Reassess your goal.** This is a great time to examine your weight-loss goals. Maybe this is your healthy weight. Or maybe this is the weight you should maintain before attempting weight loss again in a few weeks or months or even years. If so, work on keeping your weight steady, which will require continued effort. Whatever you do, don't go back to old habits. Old habits will bring back the less healthy you.

MONTH 6 ACTION STEPS

Continue your current goals or rewrite them if necessary. Additionally, select from the following goals or steps, modify them, or create your own. Choose goals from the previous weeks or last month if applicable. This month I will:

☐ Continue the following goals: _____

_____

_____

☐ Pay special attention to eliminating the saturated fat and trans fat in the food I buy.

☐ Add small amounts of avocado to my salad instead of cheese.

☐ Cook my eggs in canola oil instead of butter.

☐ Measure nuts into single serving sizes and store them in baggies.

☐ Wear my pedometer every day.

☐ Visualize the slimmer, healthier me each day before breakfast.

☐ Other: _____

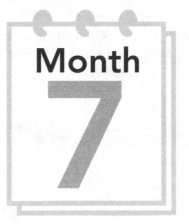

Month
7

So far, we've covered calories, carbohydrates, and fats in depth. Sodium is the focus this month. You'll understand why it can help to shake the salt habit, and you'll learn sodium-trimming strategies for the grocery store and at home.

FOR THE LONG HAUL: BE SODIUM SAVVY

Can you imagine that, centuries ago, salt was prized? Ancient Greeks used salt as currency, and Roman soldiers received it as part of their pay, giving us the word "salary." No one considered the possibility of having too much sodium. The story today is quite different. According to the *Dietary Guidelines for Americans, 2010*, African Americans, anyone age 51 years and older, and anyone with diabetes, high blood pressure, or chronic kidney disease should consume no more than 1,500 mg of sodium each day. The American Diabetes Association suggests that anyone with hypertension should keep their sodium intake to less than 1,500 mg per day. The average intake among Americans, however, is more than double that at 3,400 mg per day! Most individuals who are not in the above categories should limit sodium to 2,300 mg per day, so it seems that nearly everyone consumes too much. A high sodium intake is linked to high blood pressure, excess calcium losses in the urine, increased symptoms of heartburn, stomach cancer, and other illnesses.

So where does all this sodium come from? As a point of reference, one teaspoon of salt contains 2,325 mg of sodium. Very little of our sodium intake comes from our saltshaker, however. Most comes from restaurants and packaged foods. Limiting salt in cooking and at the table will help some but is probably not enough. You'll also need to read labels carefully (reminder: check the label for serving sizes first), seek out lower-sodium options, prepare more foods at home, fill up on vegetables and fruit, and request that restaurant chefs use little salt.

Don't let a bland or sweet taste trick you into thinking a food is low in sodium. Could you guess that a fruit Danish has more than 2 ½ times the sodium of a small order of French fries?

Food	Sodium (mg)
Fast-food grilled chicken sandwich	1,237
1 cup cottage cheese	918
1 cup reduced-sodium chicken broth	554
Fast-food chocolate shake, medium	336
Fruit Danish	333
2 tablespoons ranch dressing	328
1 slice American cheese	266
1 cup raisin bran	259
Apple cinnamon instant oatmeal	177
1 tablespoon ketchup	167
Small fries from fast-food restaurant	161
1 ounce salted peanuts	123
1 medium tomato	6
1 medium apple	2

Source: USDA Nutrient Data Laboratory
(http://www.nal.usda.gov/fnic/foodcomp/search/index.html)

TIP!

Reduced sodium does not mean low sodium. A food labeled "Low Sodium" has no more than 140 mg sodium in a standard serving. "Reduced Sodium" or "Less Sodium" indicates that the food has at least 25% less sodium than the original version of the food, but the sodium content might still be quite high. "Light in Sodium" indicates a reduction of at least 50%.

Using Less Salt at Home

Leaving higher-sodium foods on the supermarket shelves and cooking with as little salt as possible are important strategies. The following tips will help you even more.

+ Eat smaller portions of high-sodium foods.
+ Prepare your own salad dressings. To make a basic vinaigrette, mix a favorite vinegar or citrus juice with extra-virgin olive oil and seasonings. Start with a ratio of two parts oil to one part vinegar or juice, and adjust to your taste. Perhaps the simplest vinaigrette is a mix of extra-virgin olive oil, lemon juice, garlic, salt, and pepper.
+ Use only half the seasoning packet in rice mixes and other packaged foods. Better yet, prepare your rice dishes and casseroles from scratch.
+ Rinse canned beans and other vegetables.
+ Mix a can of regular vegetables or soup with a can of low-sodium vegetables or soup.
+ In recipes for bread and other baked goods, reduce the salt by ¼ to ½.
+ In other recipes, reduce the salt by at least half. In most cases, you can omit it completely. Instead, add pizzazz to your recipes with a splash of citrus juice or flavored vinegar. Experiment with herbs and spices, too. Try adding some of these herbs and spices to your dishes:
  + Basil: cheese, chicken, eggs, Italian and Mediterranean cuisines, salads, salmon, tomatoes, watermelon, zucchini
  + Cinnamon: bananas, blueberries, chicken, Middle Eastern and Moroccan cuisines
  + Dill: carrots, cucumbers, eggs, fish, potatoes, salads, tomatoes
  + Mint: carrots, cucumbers, honeydew melon, Middle Eastern cuisine, lamb, peas, salads
  + Oregano: beef, bell peppers, chicken, eggs, fish, Greek, Italian and Mediterranean cuisines, mushrooms, shrimp, tomatoes

REMEMBER YOUR PROGRESS REPORT

What changes in your health have you noticed these last several weeks? Has a recent laboratory report shown progress? Go back to your Progress Report to record all of your successes. Include how you feel, improvements in medical tests, and each new behavior that makes you proud.

MONTH 7 ACTION STEPS

Continue your current goals or rewrite them if necessary. Additionally, select from the following goals or steps, modify them, or create your own. Choose goals from the previous weeks or months if applicable. This month I will:

☐ Continue the following goals: _____

_____

_____

☐ Seek out lower-sodium options in the grocery store.

☐ Cut sodium by mixing low-sodium vegetable juice and canned vegetables with the regular versions of the products.

☐ Use herbs and spices instead of salt to season my vegetables each night at dinner.

☐ Make a vinaigrette.

☐ Start an herb garden.

☐ Record progress on my Progress Report.

☐ Increase the intensity of my workout at least twice.

☐ Other: _____

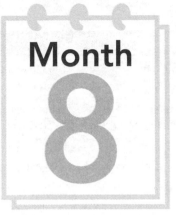

Month 8

This month we take a look at two more topics that require your attention for your entire life—your healthy heart and how to confidently say "no" to intentional or well-meaning diet saboteurs.

FOR THE LONG HAUL:
KEEP YOUR HEART HEALTHY

There is so much emphasis on weight management and blood glucose control—even in this book—that it's easy to forget that your blood pressure and cholesterol levels are equally important. People with diabetes are at a much higher risk for heart disease than individuals without diabetes, so pay as much attention to your heart health as you do your blood glucose and weight. Fortunately, the steps you take to manage one aspect of your health trickle into other areas. Being physically active helps with weight control, boosts insulin sensitivity, lowers blood pressure, and improves cholesterol levels. Losing weight improves diabetes control, blood pressure, and HDL (high-density lipoprotein or good) cholesterol levels. Trimming saturated fat from your diet can lower your LDL (low-density lipoprotein or bad) cholesterol and improve glucose control by making insulin work better. Additionally, you can help control your blood pressure by cutting back on sodium and by eating plenty of fruits and vegetables. These are all strategies we've talked about already in the book. Just take them to heart and keep working hard. And for the sake of your heart, remember to take blood pressure and cholesterol medications as prescribed by your physician.

Discuss your target blood pressure and cholesterol levels with your physician.

Ask how often you should have them measured. The ADA recommends the following targets.

Measurement	Typical Goal	Description
Blood Pressure	<130/80 mmHg	The force of blood flow inside your blood vessels
LDL Cholesterol	<100 mg/dl <70 mg/dl for those with cardiovascular disease	Sometimes called the bad cholesterol. It can cause narrowing or a blockage in the arteries.
HDL Cholesterol	>40 mg/dl for men > 50 mg/dl for women	Sometimes called the good cholesterol because it helps remove the bad cholesterol from the blood and keeps your blood vessels from getting blocked
Triglycerides	<150 mg/dl	Another type of fat in the blood that, when elevated, raises the risk for heart disease

FOR MORE INFORMATION

■ American Diabetes Association: *www.diabetes.org*
■ American Heart Association: *www.heart.org*
■ National Heart Lung and Blood Institute:
   http://www.nhlbi.nih.gov/health/public/heart/index.htm#chol

JUST SAY NO!

It's hard enough to turn down offers of your favorite foods without the extra pressure from family and friends. How can you turn down Grandma's warm-from-the-oven apple pie when she says she made it just for you? There is no easy answer for this. Clearly, however, you must keep in the forefront of your mind that your health matters, that what you eat matters, and that you matter. The tactics you use to say "no thanks" will vary depending on your situation. Some of the following may help you. Practice them before you're facing diet sabotage.

✦ Simply say "no, thank you" without an explanation. If that doesn't work, add that you're watching what you eat and thank the person for his or her understanding.
✦ Sandwich "no, thank you" between two compliments.
   ■ "It looks and smells fabulous, thanks. Too bad I'm already full. I can't wait until you make it again, though."

- ✦ Throw the blame elsewhere.
    - ▮ "I'd love to, but I promised my doctor I'd be extra careful before my next appointment."
- ✦ Ask to take some for later. You can either get rid of it or save it until a more appropriate time to eat it.
- ✦ Ask for just one bite.

- ✦ Take the food and toss it when no one is looking.
- ✦ Ask for support.
    - ▮ "I'm trying so hard to watch what I eat, and it's incredibly difficult. You can help me by not offering me snacks and sweets."

MORE FROM MARCIA C.

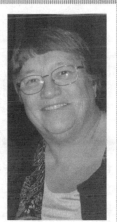

❝ It's important to get your friends and family to be your allies. Tell them you need their help. There are some diet saboteurs out there. They may not even realize that's what they are. But when they say "hey you've done so well, you deserve this treat" or "come on, it's only once in a blue moon," it's a real obstacle to losing weight and controlling blood glucose. I've discovered that the best road is to elicit their help by explaining the situation and the consequences of not following the diet plan. Giving them the chance to rise to the occasion may turn out to be a blessing for them as well. ❞

MONTH 8 ACTION STEPS

Continue your current goals or rewrite them if necessary. Additionally, select from the following goals or steps, modify them, or create your own. Choose goals from the previous weeks or months if applicable. This month I will:

☐ Continue the following goals: _____

_____

_____

☐ Ask to have a copy of my previous labs, so I know what my cholesterol and triglycerides have been. I'll keep them in a folder at home for future reference.

☐ Ask my doctor if I'm due for a blood pressure check or lab work.

☐ Imagine the situations coming up where I might be pushed to eat something I don't want or need. Practice saying "no, thank you."

☐ Continue lower-sodium cooking. Try a new low-sodium recipe.

☐ Continue to monitor my food and activity.

☐ Other: _____

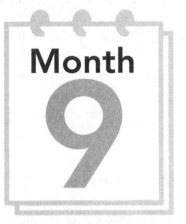

Month

9

Our food focus this month is whole grains. We'll look at what they are, how to prepare them, and what to look for on food labels. The lifelong skill that you'll practice this month is how to recognize and overcome the obstacles that tend to wreck diet and fitness plans.

FOR THE LONG HAUL: WHAT WILL YOU GAIN FROM WHOLE GRAINS

Americans eat only 15% of the recommended amount of whole grains, yet we eat 200% of the recommended limit of refined grains. Some people find whole grains scary because they don't know what to do with them. Others swear they're dry and tasteless. Most likely, they just haven't eaten whole grains that have been well prepared or seasoned. By trading in a few servings of refined grains for whole grains, you'll take in more nutrition. Other research suggests eating whole grains is linked to a reduced risk of heart disease, stroke, certain cancers, and type 2 diabetes.

WHAT ARE WHOLE GRAINS?

Whole grains include the entire grain seed: germ, bran, and endosperm. Even if the grain has been processed like it is in whole-wheat bread or whole-wheat spaghetti, it will contain all three parts of the grain. Some whole grains, like oats and brown rice, are easy to identify. Others, like whole wheat, are not so easy to identify because package labels tend to be tricky. "Made with whole grains" and "contains whole grains" are not guarantees that a product is mostly whole grain because manufacturers can make these claims even when the amount of whole grain in the product is minuscule. Look at the ingredients list to decide if the product is worth buying. If the first ingredient contains the word "whole," as in whole-wheat flour or whole-grain rye, then the product is largely whole grain. If you see "enriched wheat flour" listed first, put the product back. That's the long way to say white flour. Another method to identify whole grains is to look for the Whole Grain Stamp. If a food has a stamp on the package, it contains at least one-half serving of whole grains. Learn more about the Whole Grain Stamp at the Whole Grains Council website (*www.wholegrainscouncil.org*).

Try Some New Whole Grains

Whole Grain	Basic Instructions	Uses and Recipe Ideas
Hulled barley	Rinse first. Bring 2 cups water or broth and ½ cup barley to a boil. Simmer until tender, about 1 hour. Drain.	See Bean and Barley Salad recipe in the Appendix (page 209). Add barley to soups and stews; use instead of rice in pilafs and stir-fries.
Brown rice	Bring 1 ¼ cups water or broth and ½ cup brown rice to a boil. Simmer until the liquid is absorbed, about 45 minutes. Keep instant brown rice on hand for a quick side dish.	Use as a side dish and with stir-fries; use as a base for salads. Brown onions, mushrooms, and garlic in canola oil. Add the rice and stir. Then add the liquid and continue cooking.
Quinoa	Rinse first. Bring 1 cup water or broth and ½ cup quinoa to a boil. Simmer until tender, about 15 minutes.	See Quinoa-Stuffed Peppers recipe in the Appendix (page 218). Serve as a side dish, stuffing for poultry or vegetables, and as a base for salads. After cooking, mix with drained canned tomatoes, lime juice, and cilantro.
Wheat berries	Bring 2 cups water or broth and ½ cup wheat berries to a boil. Simmer until tender, about 1 hour. Drain.	Serve as a salad with fresh and dried fruit, herbs, nuts, and a citrus dressing.
Wild rice	Rinse first. Bring 1 ½ cups water or broth and ½ cup wild rice to a boil. Simmer until tender, about 45 minutes. Drain. Keep quick-cooking or ready-to-serve wild rice on hand for a speedy side dish.	Add to soups and use as a stuffing for poultry. Mix with diced vegetables, fruit, and herbs for a pilaf side dish.

TIP!

High fiber doesn't mean whole grain. Whole grains vary in their fiber content. Brown rice is one of the lowest in fiber, and barley is one of the highest. By eating a variety of whole grains, legumes, fruits, and vegetables, you'll get the fiber and other nutrients your body needs.

There are also plenty of high-fiber grain-based foods, such as breads, cereals, crackers, and granola bars, that are not whole grain. Instead, manufacturers added the fiber to the product. Though the fiber is important, the food is still lacking the nutrition that comes with whole grains.

OVERCOMING OBSTACLES

You will always face obstacles to eating well and taking care of yourself. Your keys to success are recognizing these hurdles and even anticipating them before they get in your way. If you're planning to celebrate a friend's birthday with a big buffet brunch, for example, you'll need to plan ahead to know which strategies you'll use to avoid overeating. Sometimes the obstacles are a little harder to anticipate, but getting in the habit of looking for potential problems will help you successfully navigate your way through them. Use the HURDLE method to overcome obstacles. The worksheet in the Appendix on page 177 will help you through each step.

HURDLE

H: How is your upcoming schedule different from your usual routine? Look ahead at your week's calendar and your day's appointments. Is there something unusual or at an unusual time?

U: Understand how any of these appointments or obligations could derail you from eating well or exercising, or otherwise get in the way of good self-care. Will they suck time out of your day or will someone else be in control of your food choices? Will you be forced to miss your favorite spin class or will you be in the car during your usual lunch hour?

R: Record your options. Brainstorm and write down every possible solution to your problem, no matter how silly it seems.

D: Decide on a solution. Review each option with an open mind. Ask yourself if you can carry it out. Do you have control, or do you need to ask for help? Is it likely to bring about the desired result?

L: List the steps you'll need to take to put the solution into practice. Know what you will do and when you will do it.

E: Exercise your choice and **Evaluate** it. Carry out your selected option. Make some notes about how well your plan worked and what you will do differently next time.

Here's an example:

H: How: Judy's daughter is in a soccer tournament. If the team continues to win, her daughter will have games every night for the next six days. Judy will know her daughter's schedule only one day in advance, and to see her daughter play, Judy may have to drive as much as an hour out of town.

U: Understand: Judy can't be certain if she'll be home for dinner any day this week.

R: Record: Judy records these options.

+ Miss the soccer games
+ Drink a meal-replacement shake and eat a piece of fruit in the car instead of eating a regular dinner
+ Pick up a fast-food dinner after checking the restaurant's nutrition information
+ Organize a "healthy" potluck with several of the other moms
+ Eat dinner very late, about 9:30
+ Pack a different dinner each night

Notice that "winging it and hoping for the best" is not one of Judy's recorded options. Judy has tried that before, and it backfired. Last year she ate whatever food was available at the soccer field or on the way to the games, which meant Judy didn't eat well that whole week.

D: Decide Judy opts for two solutions because this obstacle might continue for six days. She chooses to alternate between having a meal replacement and a piece of fruit in the car with packing a dinner she can eat at the game.

L: List Judy lists these steps in her action plan.

+ Choose an appropriate meal replacement
+ Write out menus for dinners she can pack
+ Shop for meal replacements, fruit, sandwich fixings, and other items for her bagged meal
+ Dig her extra-large lunch bag out of the hall closet
+ Be certain that her blue ice packs are kept frozen and that she returns them to the freezer each night
+ Wake up 10 minutes earlier each morning to pack her meal

E: Exercise and Evaluate: After the soccer tournament, Judy was pleased with her success, although a few nights she finished her meal feeling slightly hungry. She's already planning for next time: she'll keep some nuts or raw veggies with her in case the meal she packs isn't enough to keep her satisfied.

MONTH 9 ACTION STEPS

Continue your current goals or rewrite them if necessary. Additionally, select from the following goals or steps, modify them, or create your own. Choose goals from the previous weeks or months if applicable. This month I will:

☐ Continue the following goals: _____

_____

_____

☐ Read labels carefully to identify whole-grain products.

☐ Eat a whole grain every day at breakfast.

☐ Eat at least two servings of whole grains every day.

☐ Review my calendar for potential obstacles.

☐ Use the **HURDLE** method of problem solving.

☐ Other: _____

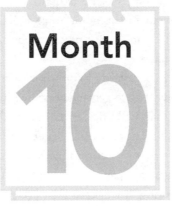

Month 10

To help you stay within your food budget, we look at strategies for making healthful eating affordable. We'll also examine one more food label trap.

FOR THE LONG HAUL: MAKING HEALTHFUL EATING AFFORDABLE

"It costs more to eat healthfully." Lots of people say this, and in some ways it's true, but not in many important ways. Yes, a salad topped with grilled chicken or salmon is more expensive than a couple of hot dogs, buns, and a plate of chips. When you look at nutritional value, however, the salad lunch is the bargain. For the extra money, you get more vitamins, minerals, fiber, protein, antioxidants, and phytochemicals and fewer fillers, additives, overly processed foods, and unhealthful fats. What's more, eating healthfully and good self-care reward you down the road with fewer health problems, fewer missed days of work, better health, and lower health care costs. This is a pay now or pay later situation. It's much better to pay now to protect your health later. This doesn't mean that you should spend your money frivolously. Being frugal is still wise, but balancing health with cost is important. These tips can help you get good nutrition without breaking the bank.

1. Prepare more meals at home. Not only will you have control over the ingredients when you cook your own food, you won't have to pay for the labor costs that come with eating at a restaurant.
2. Plan your meals by what's on sale. Before shopping, look over the supermarket flyers. If chicken is on sale, plan a few chicken meals this week.

Allow enough flexibility in your menu planning that you can swap one food for another when you see a bargain.

3. Buy in-season produce. Though it's nice to have grapes or cherries when the weather is cold, you'll pay a premium price for produce shipped from warmer climates.

4. Grow your own. A backyard or container garden is not only fun, it's also an inexpensive way to get delicious produce and herbs.

5. Shop at farmer's markets. Local, seasonal, and fresh at good prices—that's what you'll find at farmer's markets or roadside stands.

6. Join a CSA, also known as community supported agriculture. During the growing season, you'll get a big box (or two) of whatever is in season. This is how it works: a farmer sells a specified number of subscriptions and each subscriber gets a similar package. It's good for the farmer because you pay in advance, and it's good for you because of the variety and freshness of the goods you bring home each week. You will probably find yourself cooking and enjoying vegetables " you've never tried before. You can look for a CSA near you by visiting www.localharvest.org.

7. Freeze, can, or dry extra produce for later use. Freeze even small amounts of vegetables to add to casseroles and soups. Call your local USDA cooperative extension office for information on proper techniques.

8. Buy frozen fruits and vegetables. Most of the nutrients are preserved in the freezing process. Opt for the ones without added sugars and salt. If you tend to lose fruits and vegetables in the back of the refrigerator until they start to wilt or—worse—smell, buying frozen products will definitely save you money because of their long shelf life.

9. Buy generic. Store brands are often as good as or better than the pricier name brands. Compare ingredients lists and Nutrition Facts panels.

10. Search high and low. Often the least expensive items are on the top and bottom shelves because manufacturers often pay for name brand items to be at eye level.

11. Bring coupon clipping into the 21st century. Find your favorite brands on Facebook, and follow them on Twitter. You'll find some of your best deals and coupons this way.

12. Twice a week, do a 10-minute inventory of your refrigerator. Toss any vegetable that's starting to wilt into a pot of soup or add it to stews and casseroles.

13. Cut back on meat. Fill your sandwiches with 2 ounces of meat instead of 3 or 4. Split a chicken breast with a family member. Pound boneless, skinless chicken breasts before cooking to improve their taste and to make the portion look larger. Extend ground meat with lentils or chopped mushrooms.

14. Say NO to junk. Don't waste your money on food that doesn't nourish you and your family.
   ▌ Use these high-nutrition, low-cost foods: beans; lentils; white potatoes; sweet potatoes; eggs; peanut butter; canned salmon, tuna or crabmeat; oats; brown rice; barley; quinoa; frozen berries; and frozen vegetables

---

MORE FROM RUFUS G.

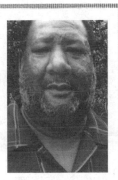

❝ Coupons are useful when I save money on things like oatmeal, whole-wheat pasta, whole-wheat bread, low-fat dairy, and fruits and vegetables. They're not usually such a good idea for over-processed foods. I used to use coupons to buy fast-food sausage and egg biscuits. I ate those biscuits nearly every day, but that's when I weighed more and had higher blood glucose and cholesterol. I hadn't eaten those sandwiches for breakfast in a long time when I got a coupon in the mail and was tempted into going back. What a waste! I saved $0.99 but filled myself with extra calories, fats, and sodium. Now I just toss those coupons in the trash. ❞

BEWARE THE HEALTH HALO

There are a lot of reasons we eat more than we realize. Brian Wansink humorously describes many of these ways in his book, *Mindless Eating: Why We Eat More Than We Think We Eat*. One trap we fall into is dubbed the "health halo." Wansink's research suggests that when people associate health benefits with a food, such as "low-fat" or "heart-healthy," they estimate that the food contains fewer calories, and, as a result, they consume more of it. Now that's definitely a problem for someone wanting to lose weight! When Wansink gave video viewers low-fat granola marked either "low-fat" or "regular" (but it was all really low fat), the people eating from the bag marked "low-fat" ate more—84 calories more.

"Low-fat" labels trick virtually everyone, but overweight people seem to be tricked more than slim individuals, according to Wansink. Heart-healthy, organic, natural, no high fructose corn syrup, whole-wheat, and other positive-sounding label terms trick shoppers with their righteous image. A whole-wheat donut is still a donut, and a soda made without high fructose corn syrup is still a soda.

So how can you guard yourself against the health halo? Your best weapon against the call of virtuous-sounding health claims is to continue to read your food labels and to weigh and measure your food.

MONTH 10 ACTION STEPS

Continue your current goals or rewrite them if necessary. Additionally, select from the following goals or steps, modify them, or create your own. Choose goals from the previous weeks or months if applicable. This month I will:

☐ Continue the following goals: _____
_____
_____

☐ Find and shop at a local farmer's market.

☐ Use Facebook and Twitter to find good deals on the brands I often buy.

☐ Try at least one generic brand food.

☐ Stock up on frozen fruits and vegetables that are on sale.

☐ Look through my pantry for foods that might have a health halo. Check the labels carefully to decide if I want to continue buying those items.

☐ Other: _____

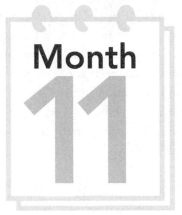

Month 11

Most people travel away from home for at least a few days each year. If you haven't traveled since you started working through this book, you probably will soon. Here are tips to help you follow or appropriately modify your plan wherever you are. As you have learned over the last 10 months, you really can enjoy treats without overindulging.

FOR THE LONG HAUL: EATING WELL WHEN AWAY FROM HOME

Traveling is another obstacle that requires you to plan ahead. (Review "Overcoming Obstacles" in Month 9 and the worksheet in the Appendix.) Often when people travel, they rationalize that because it's for just a few days or a couple of weeks, what they eat or falling off their exercise routine doesn't matter. But it does. A few extra calories here and there add up to a pound or two or three fairly quickly, especially when your physical activity drops, too. Yes, you can refocus when you get home and drop those extra pounds, but what is really important here is your mindset. Both weight control and diabetes management require lifelong effort—every day. Periodic attention won't get you very far. Try very hard not to lose sight of that. Besides, do you really want to undo any of your progress? What you've accomplished has come from hard work. Guard your new good habits; it's very hard to get back into a good routine once you've broken it. Perhaps the best plan is to follow your usual plan as closely as possible with the goal of maintaining your weight while away.

MAKE A TRAVEL PLAN

If you travel by car, pack healthful snacks in a cooler. Get plenty of ice and load up on water, vegetable juice, fresh fruit, raw colorful veggies, reduced-fat cheese, hummus, whole-grain crackers or pita bread, peanut butter sandwiches on whole-grain bread, and individual servings of reduced-fat yogurt and cottage cheese. Also, tuck a fast-food nutrition guide in your bag to help you make the best choices if you stop for a quick bite.

When traveling by plane, you don't have the luxury of a cooler, but you can toss a peanut butter sandwich, some fresh and dried fruit, and nuts into your carry-on bag.

In hotels, skip the expensive, large breakfast and enjoy some oatmeal or eggs and toast. If you have a mini-refrigerator in your room, stop by a local grocery store for some cereal, milk, and fruit. Even if breakfast comes with your room, skip the cheese Danish and choose toast, yogurt, or hot or cold cereal instead.

If you're a guest in someone else's home, let the hosts help you with your plan. Call them in advance to let them know your dietary preferences. Even if you're not expected to bring food, come with something healthful and delicious, such as a beautiful fruit bowl or a basket of goodies from a farmer's market. Offer to help prepare some meals. Stop by a nearby market to pick up a few good-for-you snacks.

Make sure to plan for the occasional treat. There's no reason to deny yourself a few extras, but plan for them and keep the portions small. If it's dessert you really want, skip the bread and pasta and share the dessert with others. If there's some high-fat favorite food on the menu, watch your fat intake for the rest of the day and allow yourself some of the food you really crave.

Look for ways to be active. Enjoy the outdoors whenever possible. Instead of sitting and reading on the beach, take a walk, play Frisbee, or collect shells. Explore local parks. Rent a bike or a canoe. When shopping or sightseeing, walk as much as you can. In hotels, take advantage of fitness centers and swimming pools, check out in-room exercise programs available on TV, pack exercise bands and a jump rope, and get on the floor for push-ups and sit-ups.

TIP!

Remember to check your blood glucose more often than usual whenever you are off your normal routine.

BE MODERATE

Throughout this book, we have talked about making lifestyle changes rather than focusing on a quick weight-loss diet or temporary food rules. Try to embrace the concept of moderation every day. Moderation implies day-to-day consistency. It also implies not depriving yourself of treats and not overindulging either. Admittedly, it's a hard concept to grasp when it comes to food and diet because we are used to messages in the media and from family telling us to strive for perfection or to feel guilty for eating cake. If you have previously followed a strict diet to lose weight and ended up regaining that weight, then you know that the all-or-nothing attitude doesn't work, even though this notion continues to make its way into diet books and TV talk shows. Instead of going to extremes, live every day near the middle. Tighten up slightly sometimes when you need to, and loosen up slightly when you can, such as on vacations. The emphasis needs to be on the word "slightly." Otherwise we're no longer talking about moderation.

MORE FROM MICHAEL B.

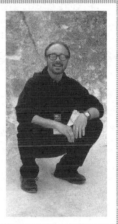

"Occasionally I want something on my "You can't have that" list. So I adjust my diet. I know if I eat a piece of candy, there has to be a tradeoff somewhere. If I overindulge and get down on myself, I know I have to get right back on the horse and keep riding."

MONTH 11 ACTION STEPS

Continue your current goals or rewrite them if necessary. Additionally, select from the following goals or steps, modify them, or create your own. Choose goals from the previous weeks or months if applicable. This month I will:

☐ Continue the following goals: _____

_____

_____

☐ Plan and purchase the food I need for traveling or for anytime I'm out of my usual routine.

☐ Review "Halt Negative Self-Talk" in Week 6 for reminders on how to avoid big setbacks.

☐ Practice fitting treats into my diet instead of leaving myself feeling either deprived or that I've overindulged.

☐ Shop for unusual fruits, vegetables, or grains.

☐ Other: _____

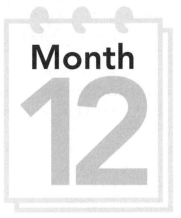

Month 12

Wow, you're approaching a year! You have covered most of the topics, skills, and strategies you need to lose weight. You have learned about diet, food, exercise, the importance of having the proper attitude, how to overcome problems, and so much more. By working through this book for a full year, you have had the opportunity to practice your new skills through each season, during holidays and vacations, when life seems simple, and when it feels much too hectic. Each chapter was designed to help you lose weight and keep it off forever. In this final chapter, we take a more focused look at strategies to help you maintain your weight loss.

MAINTAINING YOUR WEIGHT LOSS

At times, it's probably been very hard to keep focused on your plan. You will likely continue to have ups and downs. Keep resisting the lure of "breakthrough" diet plans. No doubt about it, the media and your friends will continue to announce the newest and best diet and fat-burning secrets. As you've learned over the last 11 months, there is no perfect diet for everyone and there are no secrets to fat burning, either. Eating well is not a one-size-fits-all plan. You can eat well and lose weight whether you are a vegetarian or a meat-lover, a snacker or not, a morning exerciser or an evening exerciser, or someone who quits eating at 5:00 p.m. or someone who doesn't close the kitchen until 9:00 p.m. or later.

You have lost weight this year because you've consumed fewer calories than your body burns—that is a fact. You may have done this by eating smaller portions, filling your plate with low-calorie foods, trimming fats or carbohydrates, planning your meals, counting calories or carbs, eating more vegetables, cooking more, walking instead of driving, taking exercise classes, and doing so many other things. Most successful dieters make *many* positive changes—just like the ones you have been working on all year. Hopefully, by now you are comfortable with your new diet and lifestyle. Being comfortable with it doesn't mean it is easy, however. It should be easier than it was 11 months ago, but it will probably never be effortless. If healthful eating and weight loss were easy, the entire country would be fit and slim. To maintain your weight loss, you will need to continue these new, healthier habits. Ignore the newest fad diet, no matter how tempting. Keep your ears closed to anything that sounds too good to be true. Remember that what matters is your total diet, not any one particular food. A bad diet with one or two "super foods" is still a bad diet. Likewise, a good diet with some pie now and then is still a good diet.

As we finish this year of developing new habits, it's a good time to take another look at the National Weight Control Registry (NWCR) to see the common behaviors among people who maintain their weight loss. Visit their website (*www.nwcr.ws*) for more information and to read several inspiring success stories. In fact, you can join the NWCR once you have maintained a weight loss of at least 30 pounds for one year.

Research has shown that among those who maintain their weight loss:

+ 78% eat breakfast daily.
+ 75% weigh themselves at least weekly.
+ 62% watch no more than 10 hours of television each week.
+ 90% exercise, on average, one hour per day.
+ Participants eat, on average, less than one fast-food meal each week.
+ Women's reported intake is about 1,300 calories daily, and men's reported intake is about 1,700 calories each day.
+ Only 17% consume less than 90 grams of carbohydrate daily.
+ Individuals who maintain a similar diet each day of the week and during vacations and holidays regain fewer pounds than those whose diet is inconsistent.
+ Individuals who regain the least amount of weight avoid large weight gain by weighing themselves frequently and noticing small weight gains before they become an issue.

STAY MOTIVATED

All year long, you've worked on developing knowledge, skills, and strategies. Once you have these three keys to success, they are yours. You own them, and you can rely on them. Motivation is the fourth key to success, but this one is hard to keep a strong hold on. For virtually everyone, motivation is an up-and-down phenomenon. Maintaining your motivation will sometimes be as much work as the shopping, cooking, and exercise you engage in. But it is critical to your long-term success, so learn ways to nurture your motivation along whenever you see it lagging. Lift the weight you've lost, for example. If you've dropped five pounds, pick up a five-pound sack of flour and remember what it's like to walk around with that extra weight. If you've lost 50 pounds, visit the supermarket to see 10 sacks of flour and imagine lugging them around all day.

Remember to reach for your Motivation Kit even before your motivation wanes. Continue to review your progress and make notes on your Progress Report. Jot down thoughts about how being healthier makes you feel. Be your own cheerleader and celebrate every accomplishment with at least a pat on the back. Remind yourself that every little change matters. Review various sections of this book now and then, especially the sections on beating negative self-talk, setting reasonable goals, and breaking through plateaus. Seek out the success stories of others, and visualize your own success. Buy yourself new clothes, cookware, or workout gear. Sign up for a charity walk. If you are struggling with your motivation, commit to maintaining your present weight loss. You can tend to further weight loss, if necessary, another time. Congratulations on all of your successes!

MONTH 12 ACTION STEPS

Continue your current goals or rewrite them if necessary. Additionally, select from the following goals or steps, modify them, or create your own. Choose goals from the previous weeks or months if applicable. This month I will:

☐ Continue the following goals: _____

_____

_____

☐ Visit the National Weight Control Registry website.

☐ Write an affirmation about getting back on track when I've strayed from my healthful living plan and put it in my Motivation Kit.

☐ Continue to focus on the behaviors that have brought me success: getting adequate sleep, eating breakfast, packing lunch, and

_____

_____.

☐ Review and add to my Progress Report.

☐ Mark my calendar to review strategies in this book and to add to my Progress Report at least once a month for the next year.

☐ Mark my calendar to weigh myself at least weekly.

☐ Other: _____

Appendix

WEIGHT-LOSS GRAPH AND CHART

Use this graph and chart to monitor your progress. They allow you to see the big picture rather than focusing on one or two weigh-ins.

On the chart, record your weight from your weekly weigh-ins.

Weeks

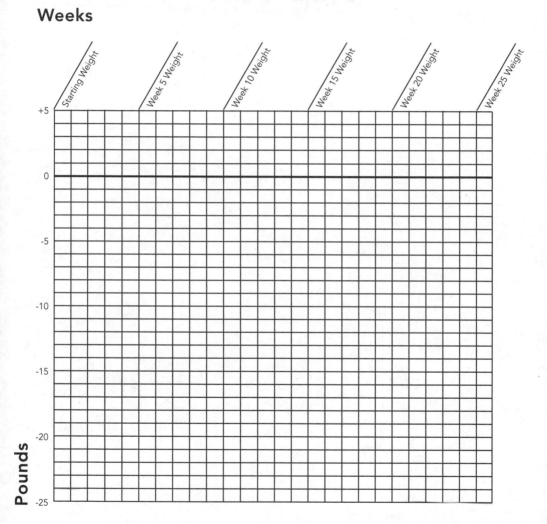

On the graph, you'll plot your weight changes over time. The numbers across the top of the graph represent weeks. The numbers down the left side represent pounds lost or gained. Mark your starting weight at the square indicating 0 pounds and Week 1. Write your weight in pounds on the line next to the number 0. Each block represents one pound. For every subsequent week, mark the appropriate square with a dot. Connect the dots, so you can see your progress.

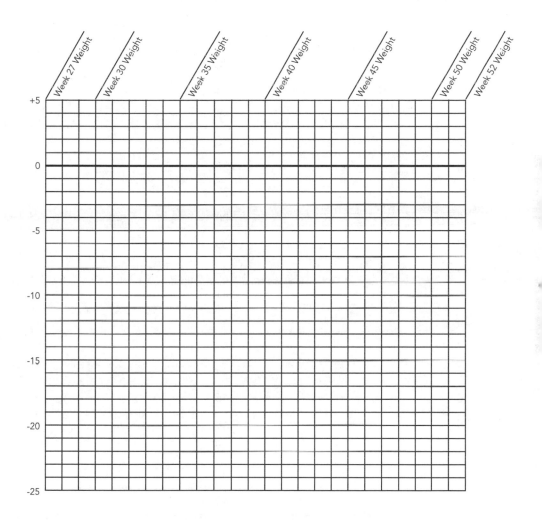

WEIGHT LOSS CHART

Week	Date	Weight	Week	Date	Weight
1			27		
2			28		
3			29		
4			30		
5			31		
6			32		
7			33		
8			34		
9			35		
10			36		
11			37		
12			38		
13			39		
14			40		
15			41		
16			42		
17			43		
18			44		
19			45		
20			46		
21			47		
22			48		
23			49		
24			50		
25			51		
26			52		

SMART GOALS WORKSHEET

Write your goals in the spaces provided. Check that it meets each of the five SMART goals principles. Then list any steps you must take to assure your success (such as get up early, grocery shop, ask for support, etc.).

S Specific:
Be specific about what you will do, how you will do it, and where you will do it. If your goal is specific, anyone who reads it will know your plan.

M Measureable:
Can you measure and objectively report your success?

A Action-oriented:
Your goal must be stated as a behavior. What action will you take?

R Realistic:
Can you achieve this goal with the resources you have and with strong effort?

T Timely:
When will you do this and when will you assess your results?

Goals:

Example:

To avoid vending machine junk at work, I will pack 5 healthy snacks on Sunday. One is for each afternoon snack break. Acceptable choices are fruit, nuts, yogurt, cottage cheese, hummus, and veggies.

S: ×　　　M: ×　　　A: ×　　　R: ×　　　T: ×

Additional steps to success: Add these foods to my shopping list. Buy them on Saturday. Prepare all 5 snacks on Sunday when I pack lunch for the next day.

1) _____

_____

_____

S: _____   M: _____   A: _____   R: _____   T: _____

Additional steps to success: _____

_____

2) _____

_____

_____

S: _____   M: _____   A: _____   R: _____   T: _____

Additional steps to success: _____

_____

3) _____

_____

_____

S: _____   M: _____   A: _____   R: _____   T: _____

Additional steps to success: _____

_____

4) _____

_____

_____

S: _____   M: _____   A: _____   R: _____   T: _____

Additional steps to success: _____

_____

FOOD RECORD

Make one copy for each day, or create your own in a notebook or on your computer.

Day: _____ Date: _____

Today's goal: _____

_____

Time/Meal (Place)	Food, Amount, Preparation	Blood Glucose, Physical Activity, & Other Notes

WEEKLY PLATE METHOD PLANNER

Use this planner to help you plan meals with lots of variety and appropriate portions.

SUNDAY		
¼ Plate Lean Meat or Other Protein	¼ Plate Grain or Starchy Vegetable	½ Plate Nonstarchy Vegetable

MONDAY		
¼ Plate Lean Meat or Other Protein	¼ Plate Grain or Starchy Vegetable	½ Plate Nonstarchy Vegetable

TUESDAY		
¼ Plate Lean Meat or Other Protein	¼ Plate Grain or Starchy Vegetable	½ Plate Nonstarchy Vegetable

WEDNESDAY		
¼ Plate Lean Meat or Other Protein	¼ Plate Grain or Starchy Vegetable	½ Plate Nonstarchy Vegetable

THURSDAY		
¼ Plate Lean Meat or Other Protein	¼ Plate Grain or Starchy Vegetable	½ Plate Nonstarchy Vegetable

FRIDAY		
¼ Plate Lean Meat or Other Protein	¼ Plate Grain or Starchy Vegetable	½ Plate Nonstarchy Vegetable

SATURDAY		
¼ Plate Lean Meat or Other Protein	¼ Plate Grain or Starchy Vegetable	½ Plate Nonstarchy Vegetable

TROUBLE TIMES AND PLACES— A RECORD

Make one copy of this record for each day or create your own version in a notebook or on your computer.

Identify those times of day or those places that make it hard to stick with your eating plan. You might include snacks, all food eaten after 5:00, all food eaten at work, food eaten alone or with others, etc. Pick what is most problematic for you.

Day: _____ Date:_____

My trouble times and places: _____

_____

Trouble Time or Place	Food, Amount, Preparation	Notes

TROUBLE FOODS—A RECORD

Make one copy of this record for each day, or create your own version in a notebook or on your computer.

Which food goals are the hardest to stick with? If you struggle to limit your soda or juice intake or to eat enough vegetables, record just beverages and vegetables. Write down and review the foods you struggle with most.

Day: _____ Date:_____

My trouble foods and goals: _____

_____

_____

_____

Trouble Food	Food, Amount, Preparation	Notes

CHECK IT

Make one copy of this form for each week, or create your own version in a notebook or on your computer.

Select as many as five goals (for example: eat breakfast, walk at lunchtime). Record your progress on a checklist. This is an objective practice; either you met your goal (ate breakfast or walked at lunchtime) or you did not.

Date:_____

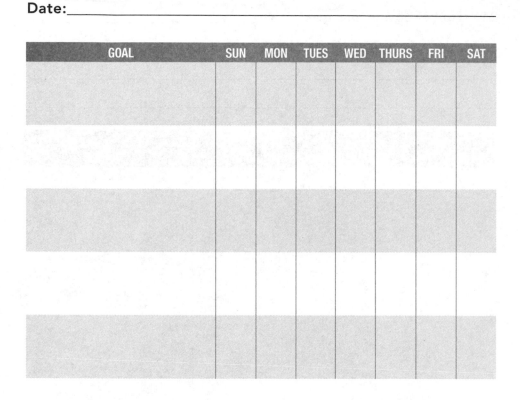

GOAL	SUN	MON	TUES	WED	THURS	FRI	SAT

Example

Date: June 3-9

GOAL	SUN	MON	TUES	WED	THURS	FRI	SAT
Eat breakfast daily	✔	✔	✔	✔	✔	✔	✔
Eat 3 cups of veggies daily	✘	✔	✔	✔	✔	✔	✘
Limit starches to one helping at dinner daily	✔	✔	✔	✔	✔	✔	✘
Exercise at least 20 minutes before work (5 days per week)	N/A	✔	✔	✔	✔	✔	N/A
Pack lunch for work (5 days per week)	N/A	✔	✔	✔	✔	✔	N/A

SCORE IT

Make one copy of this form for each week, or create your own version in a notebook or on your computer.

At the end of the day, write down a number between 1 and 10 (where 1 is very poor and 10 is excellent) to rate how successfully you have achieved your goals, such as eating appropriate portions or planning your intake ahead of time. This is a subjective score.

Date:_____

GOAL	SUN	MON	TUES	WED	THURS	FRI	SAT

Example

Date: <u>June 3-9</u>

GOAL	SUN	MON	TUES	WED	THURS	FRI	SAT
Avoid overeating	6	10	10	10	10	8	6
Plan ahead	8	10	8	10	8	7	6
Avoid too much saturated fat	7	10	10	10	9	8	8

MY PROGRESS

List each new behavior and each benefit you've gained by eating better, getting more physical activity, and paying more attention to your health. Write down every positive change you and others have noticed. Here are some examples to get you started.

- ✓ Eating smaller portions
- ✓ Not skipping meals
- ✓ Getting regular physical activity
- ✓ Better blood glucose control
- ✓ Need less blood pressure medication

- ✓ Have more energy
- ✓ Feel more confident
- ✓ No longer feel terrible remorse when I eat a bit too much
- ✓ Sleep better
- ✓ Have less knee pain

Date or Week	Progress/Benefit

OVERCOMING OBSTACLES— THE HURDLE METHOD

One key to overcoming obstacles is to anticipate them before they stand in your way. Get in the habit of using the HURDLE method to identify and prepare for problems.

H: How is your upcoming schedule different? *Think about your day, week, or month and look at your calendar. What event is unusual or scheduled for an unusual time?*

_____

_____

U: Understand how any of these appointments or obligations could derail you from eating well, exercising, or otherwise get in the way of good self-care. *Will something prevent you from eating a meal or getting to your exercise class on time? Will someone else be in charge of your meals or your schedule? How might some activity or problem prevent you from sticking to your food and exercise plan?*

_____

_____

R: Record your options. *Write down every possible solution, even if it seems silly.*

_____

_____

D: Decide on a solution. *From the list above, pick an option that is doable and likely to bring you success.*

_____

_____

L: List the steps. *Record everything you must do to make this solution work. If you must buy something, wake up early, ask for help, or prepare something, write it down.*

_____

_____

E: Exercise your choice and **Evaluate** it. *Carry out your selected option. How did it go? Would you do it this way again or make some changes? What did you learn? What will you do differently next time?*

_____

_____

SAMPLE MEAL PATTERNS FROM THE DIETARY GUIDELINES FOR AMERICANS

Remember that there is no one best diet. You and a registered dietitian can create an individualized meal plan that reflects your health, medications, schedule, food preferences, budget, and more. The *Dietary Guidelines for Americans, 2010* offers four general meal patterns that illustrate various approaches to healthful eating. You will find them on the following pages. You might also want to investigate the Mediterranean diet, discussed briefly in Week 1, as a fifth approach (visit *www.oldwayspt.org* or check out a copy of *The Mediterranean Diabetes Cookbook* by Amy Riolo to learn more). Use these approaches as additional guidance in developing your meal plan.

USDA FOOD PATTERNS

For each food group or subgroup, recommended average daily intake amounts are shown at all calorie levels. Recommended intakes from vegetable and protein subgroups are per week. For more information and tools for application, go to *ChooseMyPlate.gov*.

Calorie level of pattern	1,000	1,200	1,400	1,600	1,800	2,000	2,200	2,400	2,600	2,800	3,000	3,200
Fruits	1 c	1 c	1½ c	1½ c	1½ c	2 c	2 c	2 c	2 c	2½ c	2½ c	2½ c
Vegetables	1 c	1½ c	1½ c	2 c	2½ c	2½ c	3 c	3 c	3½ c	3½ c	4 c	4 c
Dark-green vegetables	½ c/ wk	1 c/ wk	1 c/ wk	1½ c/ wk	1½ c/ wk	1½ c/ wk	2 c/ wk	2 c/ wk	2½ c/ wk	2½ c/ wk	2½ c/ wk	2½ c/ wk
Red and orange vegetables	2½ c/ wk	3 c/ wk	3 c/ wk	4 c/ wk	5½ c/ wk	5½ c/ wk	6 c/ wk	6 c/ wk	7 c/ wk	7 c/ wk	7½ c/ wk	7½ c/ wk
Beans and peas (legumes)	½ c/ wk	½ c/ wk	½ c/ wk	1 c/ wk	1½ c/ wk	1½ c/ wk	2 c/ wk	2 c/ wk	2½ c/ wk	2½ c/ wk	3 c/ wk	3 c/ wk
Starchy vegetables	2 c/ wk	3½ c/ wk	3½ c/ wk	4 c/ wk	5 c/ wk	5 c/ wk	6 c/ wk	6 c/ wk	7 c/ wk	7 c/ wk	8 c/ wk	8 c/ wk
Other vegetables	1½ c/ wk	2½ c/ wk	2½ c/ wk	3½ c/ wk	4 c/ wk	4 c/ wk	5 c/ wk	5 c/ wk	5½ c/ wk	5½ c/ wk	7 c/ wk	7 c/ wk
Grains	3 oz-eq	4 oz-eq	5 oz-eq	5 oz-eq	6 oz-eq	6 oz-eq	7 oz-eq	8 oz-eq	9 oz-eq	10 oz-eq	10 oz-eq	10 oz-eq
Whole grains	1½ oz-eq	2 oz-eq	2½ oz-eq	3 oz-eq	3 oz-eq	3 oz-eq	3½ oz-eq	4 oz-eq	4½ oz-eq	5 oz-eq	5 oz-eq	5 oz-eq
Refined grains	1½ oz-eq	2 oz-eq	2½ oz-eq	2 oz-eq	3 oz-eq	3 oz-eq	3½ oz-eq	4 oz-eq	4½ oz-eq	5 oz-eq	5 oz-eq	5 oz-eq
Protein foods	2 oz-eq	3 oz-eq	4 oz-eq	5 oz-eq	5 oz-eq	5½ oz-eq	6 oz-eq	6½ oz-eq	6½ oz-eq	7 oz-eq	7 oz-eq	7 oz-eq
Seafood	3 oz/ wk	5 oz/ wk	6 oz/ wk	8 oz/ wk	8 oz/ wk	8 oz/ wk	9 oz/ wk	10 oz/ wk	10 oz/ wk	11 oz/ wk	11 oz/ wk	11 oz/ wk
Meat, poultry, eggs	10 oz/ wk	14 oz/ wk	19 oz/ wk	24 oz/ wk	24 oz/ wk	26 oz/ wk	29 oz/ wk	31 oz/ wk	31 oz/ wk	34 oz/ wk	34 oz/ wk	34 oz/ wk
Nuts, seeds, soy products	1 oz/ wk	2 oz/ wk	3 oz/ wk	4 oz/ wk	4 oz/ wk	4 oz/ wk	4 oz/ wk	5 oz/ wk	5 oz/ wk	5 oz/ wk	5 oz/ wk	5 oz/ wk
Dairy	2 c	2½ c	2½ c	3 c	3 c	3 c	3 c	3 c	3 c	3 c	3 c	3 c
Oils	15 g	17 g	17 g	22 g	24 g	27 g	29 g	31 g	34 g	36 g	44 g	51 g

Adapted from Dietary Guidelines for Americans, 2010.

Food group amounts are shown in cup (c) or ounce-equivalents (oz-eq). Oils are shown in grams (g). Quantity equivalents for each food group are:

Grains, 1 ounce-equivalent is: 1 one-ounce slice bread; 1 ounce uncooked pasta or rice; ½ cup cooked rice, pasta, or cereal; 1 tortilla (6" diameter); 1 pancake (5" diameter); 1 ounce ready-to-eat cereal (about 1 cup cereal flakes).

Vegetables and fruits, 1 cup equivalent is: 1 cup raw or cooked vegetable or fruit; ½ cup dried vegetable or fruit; 1 cup vegetable or fruit juice; 2 cups leafy salad greens.

Protein foods, 1 ounce-equivalent is: 1 ounce lean meat, poultry, seafood; 1 egg; 1 Tbsp peanut butter; ½ ounce nuts or seeds. Also, ¼ cup cooked beans or peas may be counted as 1 ounce-equivalent.

Dairy, 1 cup equivalent is: 1 cup milk, fortified soy beverage, or yogurt; 1½ ounces natural cheese (e.g., cheddar); 2 ounces of processed cheese (e.g., American).

LACTO-OVO VEGETARIAN ADAPTATION OF THE USDA FOOD PATTERNS

For each food group or subgroup, recommended average daily intake amounts are shown at all calorie levels. Recommended intakes from vegetable and protein subgroups are per week. For more information and tools for application, go to *ChooseMyPlate.gov*.

Calorie level of pattern	1,000	1,200	1,400	1,600	1,800	2,000	2,200	2,400	2,600	2,800	3,000	3,200
Fruits	1 c	1 c	1½ c	1½ c	1½ c	2 c	2 c	2 c	2 c	2½ c	2½ c	2½ c
Vegetables	1 c	1½ c	1½ c	2 c	2½ c	2½ c	3 c	3 c	3½ c	3½ c	4 c	4 c
Dark-green vegetables	½ c/wk	1 c/wk	1 c/wk	1½ c/wk	1½ c/wk	1½ c/wk	2 c/wk	2 c/wk	2½ c/wk	2½ c/wk	2½ c/wk	2½ c/wk
Red and orange vegetables	2½ c/wk	3 c/wk	3 c/wk	4 c/wk	5½ c/wk	5½ c/wk	6 c/wk	6 c/wk	7 c/wk	7 c/wk	7½ c/wk	7½ c/wk
Beans and peas (legumes)	½ c/wk	½ c/wk	½ c/wk	1 c/wk	1½ c/wk	1½ c/wk	2 c/wk	2 c/wk	2½ c/wk	2½ c/wk	3 c/wk	3 c/wk
Starchy vegetables	2 c/wk	3½ c/wk	3½ c/wk	4 c/wk	5 c/wk	5 c/wk	6 c/wk	6 c/wk	7 c/wk	7 c/wk	8 c/wk	8 c/wk
Other vegetables	1½ c/wk	2½ c/wk	2½ c/wk	3½ c/wk	4 c/wk	4 c/wk	5 c/wk	5 c/wk	5½ c/wk	5½ c/wk	7 c/wk	7 c/wk
Grains	3 oz-eq	4 oz-eq	5 oz-eq	5 oz-eq	6 oz-eq	6 oz-eq	7 oz-eq	8 oz-eq	9 oz-eq	10 oz-eq	10 oz-eq	10 oz-eq
Whole grains	1½ oz-eq	2 oz-eq	2½ oz-eq	3 oz-eq	3 oz-eq	3 oz-eq	3½ oz-eq	4 oz-eq	4½ oz-eq	5 oz-eq	5 oz-eq	5 oz-eq
Refined grains	1½ oz-eq	2 oz-eq	2½ oz-eq	2 oz-eq	3 oz-eq	3 oz-eq	3½ oz-eq	4 oz-eq	4½ oz-eq	5 oz-eq	5 oz-eq	5 oz-eq
Protein foods	2 oz-eq	3 oz-eq	4 oz-eq	5 oz-eq	5 oz-eq	5½	6 oz-eq	6½	6½	7 oz-eq	7 oz-eq	7 oz-eq
Eggs	1 oz-eq/wk	2 oz-eq/wk	3 oz-eq/wk	4 oz-eq/wk	4 oz-eq/wk	4 oz-eq/wk	4 oz-eq/wk	5 oz-eq/wk	5 oz-eq/wk	5 oz-eq/wk	5 oz-eq/wk	5 oz-eq/wk
Beans and peas	3½ oz-eq/wk	5 oz-eq/wk	7 oz-eq/wk	9 oz-eq/wk	9 oz-eq/wk	10 oz-eq/wk	10 oz-eq/wk	11 oz-eq/wk	11 oz-eq/wk	12 oz-eq/wk	12 oz-eq/wk	12 oz-eq/wk
Soy products	4 oz-eq/wk	6 oz-eq/wk	8 oz-eq/wk	11 oz-eq/wk	11 oz-eq/wk	12 oz-eq/wk	13 oz-eq/wk	14 oz-eq/wk	14 oz-eq/wk	15 oz-eq/wk	15 oz-eq/wk	15 oz-eq/wk
Nuts and seeds	5 oz-eq/wk	7 oz-eq/wk	10 oz-eq/wk	12 oz-eq/wk	12 oz-eq/wk	13 oz-eq/wk	15 oz-eq/wk	16 oz-eq/wk	16 oz-eq/wk	17 oz-eq/wk	17 oz-eq/wk	17 oz-eq/wk
Dairy	2 c	2½ c	2½ c	3 c	3 c	3 c	3 c	3 c	3 c	3 c	3 c	3 c
Oils	12 g	13 g	12 g	15 g	17 g	19 g	21 g	22 g	25 g	26 g	34 g	41 g

Adapted from Dietary Guidelines for Americans, 2010.

Food group amounts are shown in cup (c) or ounce-equivalents (oz-eq). Oils are shown in grams (g). Quantity equivalents for each food group are:

Grains, 1 ounce-equivalent is: 1 one-ounce slice bread; 1 ounce uncooked pasta or rice; ½ cup cooked rice, pasta, or cereal; 1 tortilla (6" diameter); 1 pancake (5" diameter); 1 ounce ready-to-eat cereal (about 1 cup cereal flakes).

Vegetables and fruits, 1 cup equivalent is: 1 cup raw or cooked vegetable or fruit; ½ cup dried vegetable or fruit; 1 cup vegetable or fruit juice; 2 cups leafy salad greens.

Protein foods, 1 ounce-equivalent is: 1 ounce lean meat, poultry, seafood; 1 egg; 1 Tbsp peanut butter; ½ ounce nuts or seeds. Also, ¼ cup cooked beans or peas may be counted as 1 ounce-equivalent.

Dairy, 1 cup equivalent is: 1 cup milk, fortified soy beverage, or yogurt; 1½ ounces natural cheese (e.g., cheddar); 2 ounces of processed cheese (e.g., American).

VEGAN ADAPTATION OF THE USDA FOOD PATTERNS

For each food group or subgroup, recommended average daily intake amounts are shown at all calorie levels. Recommended intakes from vegetable and protein subgroups are per week. For more information and tools for application, go to *ChooseMyPlate.gov.*

Calorie level of pattern	1,000	1,200	1,400	1,600	1,800	2,000	2,200	2,400	2,600	2,800	3,000	3,200
Fruits	1 c	1 c	1½ c	1½ c	1½ c	2 c	2 c	2 c	2 c	2½ c	2½ c	2½ c
Vegetables	1 c	1½ c	1½ c	2 c	2½ c	2½ c	3 c	3 c	3½ c	3½ c	4 c	4 c
Dark-green vegetables	½ c/wk	1 c/wk	1 c/wk	1½ c/wk	1½ c/wk	1½ c/wk	2 c/wk	2 c/wk	2½ c/wk	2½ c/wk	2½ c/wk	2½ c/wk
Red and orange vegetables	2½ c/wk	3 c/wk	3 c/wk	4 c/wk	5½ c/wk	5½ c/wk	6 c/wk	6 c/wk	7 c/wk	7 c/wk	7½ c/wk	7½ c/wk
Beans and peas (legumes)	½ c/wk	½ c/wk	½ c/wk	1 c/wk	1½ c/wk	1½ c/wk	2 c/wk	2 c/wk	2½ c/wk	2½ c/wk	3 c/wk	3 c/wk
Starchy vegetables	2 c/wk	3½ c/wk	3½ c/wk	4 c/wk	5 c/wk	5 c/wk	6 c/wk	6 c/wk	7 c/wk	7 c/wk	8 c/wk	8 c/wk
Other vegetables	1½ c/wk	2½ c/wk	2½ c/wk	3½ c/wk	4 c/wk	4 c/wk	5 c/wk	5 c/wk	5½ c/wk	5½ c/wk	7 c/wk	7 c/wk
Grains	3 oz-eq	4 oz-eq	5 oz-eq	5 oz-eq	6 oz-eq	6 oz-eq	7 oz-eq	8 oz-eq	9 oz-eq	10 oz-eq	10 oz-eq	10 oz-eq
Whole grains	1½ oz-eq	2 oz-eq	2½ oz-eq	3 oz-eq	3 oz-eq	3 oz-eq	3½	4 oz-eq	4½	5 oz-eq	5 oz-eq	5 oz-eq
Refined grains	1½ oz-eq	2 oz-eq	2½ oz-eq	2 oz-eq	3 oz-eq	3 oz-eq	3½ oz-eq	4 oz-eq	4½ oz-eq	5 oz-eq	5 oz-eq	5 oz-eq
Protein foods	2 oz-eq	3 oz-eq	4 oz-eq	5 oz-eq	5 oz-eq	5½ oz-eq	6 oz-eq	6½ oz-eq	6½ oz-eq	7 oz-eq	7 oz-eq	7 oz-eq
Beans and peas	5 oz-eq/wk	7 oz-eq/wk	10 oz-eq/wk	12 oz-eq/wk	12 oz-eq/wk	13 oz-eq/wk	15 oz-eq/wk	16 oz-eq/wk	16 oz-eq/wk	17 oz-eq/wk	17 oz-eq/wk	17 oz-eq/wk
Soy products	4 oz-eq/wk	5 oz-eq/wk	7 oz-eq/wk	9 oz-eq/wk	9 oz-eq/wk	10 oz-eq/wk	11 oz-eq/wk	11 oz-eq/wk	11 oz-eq/wk	12 oz-eq/wk	12 oz-eq/wk	12 oz-eq/wk
Nuts and seeds	6 oz-eq/wk	8 oz-eq/wk	11 oz-eq/wk	14 oz-eq/wk	14 oz-eq/wk	15 oz-eq/wk	17 oz-eq/wk	18 oz-eq/wk	18 oz-eq/wk	20 oz-eq/wk	20 oz-eq/wk	20 oz-eq/wk
Dairy	2 c	2½ c	2½ c	3 c	3 c	3 c	3 c	3 c	3 c	3 c	3 c	3 c
Oils	12 g	12 g	11 g	14 g	16 g	18 g	20 g	21 g	24 g	25 g	33 g	40 g

Adapted from Dietary Guidelines for Americans, 2010.

Food group amounts are shown in cup (c) or ounce-equivalents (oz-eq). Oils are shown in grams (g). Quantity equivalents for each food group are:

Grains, 1 ounce-equivalent is: 1 one-ounce slice bread; 1 ounce uncooked pasta or rice; ½ cup cooked rice, pasta, or cereal; 1 tortilla (6" diameter); 1 pancake (5" diameter); 1 ounce ready-to-eat cereal (about 1 cup cereal flakes).

Vegetables and fruits, 1 cup equivalent is: 1 cup raw or cooked vegetable or fruit; ½ cup dried vegetable or fruit; 1 cup vegetable or fruit juice; 2 cups leafy salad greens.

Protein foods, 1 ounce-equivalent is: 1 ounce lean meat, poultry, seafood; 1 egg; 1 Tbsp peanut butter; ½ ounce nuts or seeds. Also, ¼ cup cooked beans or peas may be counted as 1 ounce-equivalent.

Dairy, 1 cup equivalent is: 1 cup milk, fortified soy beverage, or yogurt; 1½ ounces natural cheese (e.g., cheddar); 2 ounces of processed cheese (e.g., American).

THE DASH (DIETARY APPROACHES TO STOP HYPERTENSION) EATING PLAN

The number of daily servings in a food group varies depending on caloric needs.

Food Group	1,200 cal	1,400 cal	1,600 cal	1,800 cal	2,000 cal	2,600 cal	3,100 cal	Serving Sizes
Grains	4–5	5–6	6	6	6–8	10–11	12–13	1 slice bread 1 oz dry cereal ½ cup cooked rice, pasta, or cereal
Vegetables	3–4	3–4	3–4	4–5	4–5	5–6	6	1 cup raw leafy vegetables ½ cup cut-up raw or cooked vegetables ½ cup vegetable juice
Fruits	3–4	4	4	4–5	4–5	5–6	6	1 medium fruit ¼ cup dried fruit ½ cup fresh, frozen, or canned fruit ½ cup fruit juice
Fat-free or low-fat milk and milk products	2–3	2–3	2–3	2–3	2–3	3	3–4	1 cup milk or yogurt 1½ oz cheese
Lean meats, poultry, and fish	3 or less	3–4 or less	3–4 or less	6 or less	6 or less	6 or less	6–9	1 oz cooked meats, poultry, or fish 1 egg
Nuts, seeds, and legumes	3 per week	3 per week	3–4 per week	4 per week	4–5 per week	1	1	⅓ cup or 1½ oz nuts 2 Tbsp peanut butter 2 Tbsp or ½ oz seeds ½ cup cooked legumes (dried beans, peas)
Fats and oils	1	1	2	2–3	2–3	3	4	1 tsp soft margarine 1 tsp vegetable oil 1 Tbsp mayonnaise 1 Tbsp salad dressing
Sweets and added sugars	3 or less per week	3 or less per week	3 or less per week	5 or less per week	5 or less per week	<2	<2	1 Tbsp sugar 1 Tbsp jelly or jam ½ cup sorbet, gelatin dessert 1 cup lemonade
Maximum sodium limit	2,300 mg/day	2,300 mg/day	2,300 mg/day	2,300 mg/day	2,300 mg/day	2,300 mg/day	2,300 mg/day	

7-DAY MENUS

Use these menus as a guide and as inspiration. There is no reason to think that you will like each of the items on these menus or that they include foods that are in season and readily available. Additionally, they may contain more or less carbohydrate than the amount you need, and they may suggest more or fewer snacks than you prefer. There is nothing magical about them. They are here simply to help you learn to plan your meals and expand your usual food choices. Please adapt them at will.

You will notice that a nutritional analysis accompanies each meal and snack. These numbers are ballpark figures only. There is significant nutrient variation in packaged foods from brand to brand and even within brands. Fresh produce varies considerably as well. The nutritional content of an apple, for example, depends on the time of year it was grown and harvested, the amount of sunlight and rain, the soil in which it was grown, and more.

DAY 1
1,300 Calories

Meal/Snack Nutrition Data	Menu
Breakfast Calories 311 Fat 13g Saturated Fat 3g Sodium 375mg Carbohydrate 27g Fiber 2g Protein 21g	2 medium eggs with ½ cup sautéed baby spinach and ¼ cup diced tomatoes, prepared in 1 tsp canola oil 1 medium Clementine 1 cup nonfat milk
Morning Snack Calories Fat Saturated Fat Sodium Carbohydrate Fiber Protein	None
Lunch Calories 245 Fat 5g Saturated Fat 1g Sodium 678mg Carbohydrate 37g Fiber 12g Protein 19g	Turkey sandwich: 2 oz reduced-sodium turkey breast with tomatoes, cucumbers, lettuce, 2 tsp light mayonnaise and mustard on 2 slices light, high-fiber whole-wheat bread 1¼ cups whole strawberries
Afternoon Snack Calories 177 Fat 8g Saturated Fat 1g Sodium 61mg Carbohydrate 24g Fiber 5g Protein 4g	1 small sliced apple with 1 Tbsp natural peanut butter
Dinner Calories 582 Fat 18g Saturated Fat 3g Sodium 1,146mg Carbohydrate 60g Fiber 10g Protein 50g	1 serving Fish en Papillote 2 cups salad with romaine lettuce and 2 Tbsp reduced-fat red wine vinaigrette ⅔ cup wild rice 1 cup cooked chopped broccoli 1 Tbsp reduced-calorie vegetable oil spread shared between the rice and broccoli 1 cup nonfat milk

DAY 1
1,800 Calories

Meal/Snack Nutrition Data	Menu
Breakfast Calories 418 Fat 15g Saturated Fat 3g Sodium 482mg Carbohydrate 58g Fiber 14g Protein 27g	2 medium eggs with ½ cup sautéed baby spinach and ¼ cup diced tomatoes, prepared in 1 tsp canola oil 1 medium Clementine 1 cup nonfat milk ⅔ cup All-Bran cereal
Morning Snack Calories Fat Saturated Fat Sodium Carbohydrate Fiber Protein	None
Lunch Calories 460 Fat 13g Saturated Fat 4g Sodium 1,088mg Carbohydrate 52g Fiber 9g Protein 37g	Turkey sandwich: 3 oz reduced-sodium turkey breast with 1 oz 50% reduced-fat jalapeño cheddar cheese, tomatoes, cucumbers, lettuce, 1 Tbsp light mayonnaise and mustard on 2 slices 100% whole-wheat bread 1¼ cups whole strawberries
Afternoon Snack Calories 264 Fat 15g Saturated Fat 3g Sodium 93mg Carbohydrate 29g Fiber 7g Protein 8g	1 medium apple 1 oz dry-roasted, no-salt-added peanuts
Dinner Calories 665 Fat 19g Saturated Fat 3g Sodium 1,180mg Carbohydrate 77g Fiber 13g Protein 54g	1 serving Fish en Papillote 2 cups salad with romaine lettuce and 2 Tbsp reduced-fat red wine vinaigrette 1 cup wild rice 1½ cups cooked chopped broccoli 1 Tbsp reduced-calorie vegetable oil spread shared between the rice and broccoli 1 cup nonfat milk (can be saved for evening snack)

DAY 2
1,300 Calories

Meal/Snack Nutrition Data	Menu
Breakfast Calories 203 Fat 0g Saturated Fat 0g Sodium 101mg Carbohydrate 30g Fiber 5g Protein 22g	1 serving Mixed Berry Smoothie
Morning Snack Calories 121 Fat 7g Saturated Fat 1g Sodium 0mg Carbohydrate 11g Fiber 2g Protein 3g	25 pistachios in the shell 2 fresh apricots
Lunch Calories 413 Fat 13g Saturated Fat 2g Sodium 1,406mg Carbohydrate 42g Fiber 6g Protein 35g	Grilled chicken salad: 2 cups romaine lettuce, chopped red bell pepper, and red onion, 3 oz grilled chicken breast, and 2 Tbsp light ranch dressing 1 cup Rita's New England Clam Chowder 10 Triscuit Thin Crisp crackers
Afternoon Snack Calories 125 Fat 5g Saturated Fat 3g Sodium 170mg Carbohydrate 16g Fiber 1g Protein 9g	17 purple grapes 1 oz 50% reduced-fat cheddar cheese
Dinner Calories 398 Fat 14g Saturated Fat 3g Sodium 312mg Carbohydrate 57g Fiber 13g Protein 16g	2 halves Quinoa-Stuffed Peppers ½ cup steamed carrot slices with 2 tsp reduced-calorie vegetable oil spread
Evening Snack Calories Fat Saturated Fat Sodium Carbohydrate Fiber Protein	None

DAY 2
1,800 Calories

Meal/Snack Nutrition Data	Menu
Breakfast Calories 383 Fat 9g Saturated Fat 1g Sodium 226mg Carbohydrate 51g Fiber 8g Protein 29g	1 serving Mixed Berry Smoothie 1 slice whole-grain cinnamon raisin bread 1 Tbsp natural peanut butter
Morning Snack Calories 199 Fat 14g Saturated Fat 2g Sodium 0mg Carbohydrate 15g Fiber 4g Protein 6g	49 pistachios in the shell 2 fresh apricots
Lunch Calories 523 Fat 16g Saturated Fat 3g Sodium 1,727mg Carbohydrate 53g Fiber 7g Protein 45g	Grilled chicken salad: 2 cups romaine lettuce, chopped red bell pepper, and red onion, 4 oz grilled chicken breast, and 2 Tbsp light ranch dressing 1¼ cups Rita's New England Clam Chowder 15 Triscuit Thin Crisp crackers
Afternoon Snack Calories 125 Fat 5g Saturated Fat 3g Sodium 170mg Carbohydrate 16g Fiber 1g Protein 9g	17 purple grapes 1 oz 50% reduced-fat cheddar cheese
Dinner Calories 426 Fat 14g Saturated Fat 3g Sodium 357mg Carbohydrate 63mg Fiber 16g Protein 16g	2 halves Quinoa-Stuffed Peppers 1 cup steamed carrot slices with 2 tsp reduced-calorie vegetable oil spread
Evening Snack Calories 90 Fat 0g Saturated Fat 0g Sodium 130mg Carbohydrate 13g Fiber 0g Protein 9g	1 cup nonfat milk

DAY 3
1,300 Calories

Meal/Snack Nutrition Data	Menu
Breakfast Calories 272 Fat 3g Saturated Fat 1g Sodium 365mg Carbohydrate 47g Fiber 4g Protein 16g	½ Breakfast Pizza (½ English muffin) ½ mango 1 cup nonfat milk
Morning Snack Calories 127 Fat 11g Saturated Fat 2g Sodium 68mg Carbohydrate 3g Fiber 2g Protein 6g	¾ oz oil-roasted peanuts
Lunch Calories 447 Fat 25g Saturated Fat 4g Sodium 591mg Carbohydrate 40 Fiber 8g Protein 21g	Large mixed salad: 2 cups romaine lettuce, ½ cup cherry tomatoes, 1 chopped carrot, 1 oz avocado, 2 Tbsp sunflower seeds, 1 hard-boiled egg, ¼ cup low-fat shredded cheddar cheese, and 2 Tbsp light French dressing 1 cup cantaloupe cubes
Afternoon Snack Calories 100 Fat 0g Saturated Fat 0g Sodium 85mg Carbohydrate 19g Fiber 0g Protein 5g	6 oz flavored, artificially sweetened nonfat yogurt, such as Yoplait Light Key Lime Pie
Dinner Calories 430 Fat 11g Saturated Fat 3g Sodium 735mg Carbohydrate 55g Fiber 9g Protein 28g	1 serving Soft Turkey Tacos 2 Tbsp salsa

DAY 3
1,800 Calories

Meal/Snack Nutrition Data	Menu
Breakfast Calories 385 Fat 6g Saturated Fat 2g Sodium 599mg Carbohydrate 64g Fiber 7g Protein 22g	1 Breakfast Pizza (1 whole English muffin) ½ mango 1 cup nonfat milk
Morning Snack Calories 185 Fat 18g Saturated Fat 2g Sodium 1mg Carbohydrate 4g Fiber 2g Protein 4g	1 oz walnuts
Lunch Calories 665 Fat 34g Saturated Fat 6g Sodium 1,224mg Carbohydrate 57g Fiber 12g Protein 42g	Large mixed salad: 2 cups romaine lettuce, ½ cup cherry tomatoes, 1 chopped carrot, 2 ounces avocado, 2 Tbsp sunflower seeds, 1 hard-boiled egg, ¼ cup low-fat shredded cheddar cheese, 3 oz reduced-sodium turkey breast, and 2 Tbsp light French dressing 1 cup cantaloupe cubes 10 Triscuit Thin Crisp crackers
Afternoon Snack Calories 154 Fat 1g Saturated Fat 0g Sodium 139mg Carbohydrate 34g Fiber 6g Protein 8g	6 oz flavored, artificially sweetened nonfat yogurt, such as Yoplait Light Key Lime Pie ⅓ cup All-Bran cereal
Dinner Calories 430 Fat 11g Saturated Fat 3g Sodium 735mg Carbohydrate 55g Fiber 9g Protein 28g	1 serving Soft Turkey Tacos 2 Tbsp salsa

DAY 4
1,300 Calories

Meal/Snack Nutrition Data	Menu
Breakfast Calories 228 Fat 9 Saturated Fat 1g Sodium 99mg Carbohydrate 34g Fiber 5g Protein 7g	1 slice whole-grain cinnamon raisin bread 1 Tbsp almond butter ½ medium (about 7½ inches) banana
Morning Snack Calories Fat Saturated Fat Sodium Carbohydrate Fiber Protein	None
Lunch Calories 303 Fat 5g Saturated Fat 1g Sodium 363mg Carbohydrate 57g Fiber 17g Protein 13g	1 cup Vegetarian Chili 1 Tbsp shredded reduced-fat sharp cheddar cheese 1 small apple
Afternoon Snack Calories Fat Saturated Fat Sodium Carbohydrate Fiber Protein	None
Dinner Calories 606 Fat 30g Saturated Fat 6g Sodium 645mg Carbohydrate 46g Fiber 8g Protein 42g	1 serving Asian Salmon ⅔ cup whole-wheat pasta with 1 tsp reduced-calorie vegetable oil spread 10 medium asparagus spears, roasted with 1 tsp olive oil 1 cup nonfat milk
Evening Snack Calories 163 Fat 6g Saturated Fat 2g Sodium 147mg Carbohydrate 19g Fiber 1g Protein 10g	4 chocolate-covered almonds 1 cup nonfat milk

DAY 4
1,800 Calories

Meal/Snack Nutrition Data	Menu
Breakfast Calories 404 Fat 18g Saturated Fat 1g Sodium 197mg Carbohydrate 55g Fiber 9g Protein 13g	2 slices whole-grain cinnamon raisin bread 2 Tbsp almond butter ½ medium (about 7½ inches) banana
Morning Snack Calories Fat Saturated Fat Sodium Carbohydrate Fiber Protein	None
Lunch Calories 420 Fat 11g Saturated Fat 4g Sodium 701mg Carbohydrate 63g Fiber 21g Protein 23g	1½ cup Vegetarian Chili 3 Tbsp shredded reduced-fat sharp cheddar cheese 6 Triscuit Thin Crisps
Afternoon Snack Calories 228 Fat 1g Saturated Fat 0g Sodium 112mg Carbohydrate 32g Fiber 6g Protein 24g	1¼ cups whole strawberries 1 cup nonfat plain Greek yogurt ¼ cup Go Lean Crunch cereal
Dinner Calories 601 Fat 33g Saturated Fat 6g Sodium 554mg Carbohydrate 47g Fiber 11g Protein 36g	1 serving Asian Salmon 1 cup whole-wheat pasta with 2 tsp reduced-calorie vegetable oil spread 12 medium asparagus spears, roasted with 1 tsp olive oil
Evening Snack Calories 200 Fat 9g Saturated Fat 3g Sodium 155mg Carbohydrate 22g Fiber 2g Protein 11g	6 chocolate-covered almonds 1 cup nonfat milk

DAY 5
1,300 Calories

Meal/Snack Nutrition Data	Menu
Breakfast Calories 364 Fat 7g Saturated Fat 3g Sodium 852mg Carbohydrate 51g Fiber 8g Protein 30g	1 cup 2% fat cottage cheese 1 cup blueberries ½ cup Go Lean Crunch cereal
Morning Snack Calories Fat Saturated Fat Sodium Carbohydrate Fiber Protein	None
Lunch Calories 316 Fat 10g Saturated Fat 2g Sodium 242mg Carbohydrate 53g Fiber 11g Protein 8g	1⅓ cups Bean and Barley Salad 1 small pear
Afternoon Snack Calories Fat Saturated Fat Sodium Carbohydrate Fiber Protein	None
Dinner Calories 591 Fat 19g Saturated Fat 5g Sodium 474mg Carbohydrate 55g Fiber 7g Protein 51g	4 oz top sirloin steak, trimmed of fat and broiled 1 small baked potato with 2 tsp reduced-calorie vegetable oil spread and 1 Tbsp chopped chives 1 tomato, sliced ⅔ cup Lemon-Spiked Roasted Cauliflower 1 cup nonfat milk

DAY 5
1,800 Calories

Meal/Snack Nutrition Data	Menu
Breakfast Calories 398 Fat 8g Saturated Fat 3g Sodium 869mg Carbohydrate 57g Fiber 9g Protein 31g	1 cup 2% fat cottage cheese 1 cup blueberries 2/3 cup Go Lean Crunch cereal
Morning Snack Calories 263 Fat 19g Saturated Fat 2g Sodium 2mg Carbohydrate 24g Fiber 5g Protein 5g	1 small apple 1 oz walnuts
Lunch Calories 316 Fat 10g Saturated Fat 2g Sodium 242mg Carbohydrate 53g Fiber 11g Protein 8g	1 1/3 cups Bean and Barley Salad 1 small pear
Afternoon Snack Calories 183 Fat 6g Saturated Fat 2g Sodium 787mg Carbohydrate 32g Fiber 5g Protein 5g	1 oz baked tortilla chips 3 Tbsp guacamole 3 Tbsp salsa
Dinner Calories 669 Fat 24g Saturated Fat 6g Sodium 525mg Carbohydrate 55g Fiber 7g Protein 58g	5 oz top sirloin steak, broiled and trimmed of fat 1 small baked potato with 1 Tbsp reduced-calorie vegetable oil spread and 1 Tbsp chopped chives 1 tomato, sliced 2/3 cup Lemon-Spiked Roasted Cauliflower 1 cup nonfat milk

DAY 6
1,300 Calories

Meal/Snack Nutrition Data	Menu
Breakfast Calories 398 Fat 13g Saturated Fat 1g Sodium 131mg Carbohydrate 55g Fiber 11g Protein 18g	¼ cup dry steel-cut oats prepared with water according to package directions ½ medium (about 7½ inches) banana 2 Tbsp chopped walnuts 1 cup nonfat milk
Morning Snack Calories Fat Saturated Fat Sodium Carbohydrate Fiber Protein	None
Lunch Calories 372 Fat 11g Saturated Fat 2g Sodium 875mg Carbohydrate 48g Fiber 7g Protein 20g	1 slice Judy's Lightened Meatloaf 1⅛ cups Veggie-Packed Potato Salad 1 tomato, sliced, drizzled with balsamic vinegar
Afternoon Snack Calories 60 Fat 0g Saturated Fat 0g Sodium 0mg Carbohydrate 15g Fiber 2g Protein 1g	1 medium peach
Dinner Calories 564 Fat 22g Saturated Fat 6g Sodium 983mg Carbohydrate 58g Fiber 8g Protein 38g	¼ recipe Sautéed Scallops 1½ cups spring lettuce mix with 1 Tbsp dried cranberries, 1 oz soft goat cheese, 1 Tbsp chopped pecans, and 2 Tbsp fat-free raspberry vinaigrette ½ cup wild rice 1 cup sautéed spinach prepared with 1 tsp olive oil and garlic 1 cup nonfat milk
Evening Snack Calories Fat Saturated Fat Sodium Carbohydrate Fiber Protein	None

DAY 6
1,800 Calories

Meal/Snack Nutrition Data	Menu
Breakfast Calories 398 Fat 13g Saturated Fat 1g Sodium 131mg Carbohydrate 55g Fiber 11g Protein 18g	¼ cup dry steel-cut oats prepared with water according to package directions ½ medium (about 7½ inches) banana 2 Tbsp chopped walnuts 1 cup nonfat milk
Morning Snack Calories 118 Fat 5g Saturated Fat 0g Sodium 284mg Carbohydrate 17g Fiber 4g Protein 3g	3 Tbsp hummus with ½ red bell pepper, sliced, and 1 carrot, cut into sticks
Lunch Calories 462 Fat 13g Saturated Fat 3g Sodium 1,126mg Carbohydrate 58g Fiber 9g Protein 28g	1½ slices Judy's Lightened Meatloaf 1⅛ cups Veggie-Packed Potato Salad 1 tomato, sliced, drizzled with balsamic vinegar
Afternoon Snack Calories 180 Fat 0g Saturated Fat 0g Sodium 85mg Carbohydrate 24g Fiber 2g Protein 21g	1 medium peach 1 cup nonfat Greek yogurt
Dinner Calories 604 Fat 27g Saturated Fat 7g Sodium 855mg Carbohydrate 64g Fiber 10g Protein 33g	¼ recipe Sautéed Scallops 1½ cups spring lettuce mix with 1 Tbsp dried cranberries, 1 oz soft goat cheese, 2 Tbsp chopped pecans, and 2 Tbsp fat-free raspberry vinaigrette 1 cup wild rice 1 cup sautéed spinach prepared with 1 tsp olive oil and garlic
Evening Snack Calories 90 Fat 0g Saturated Fat 0g Sodium 130mg Carbohydrate 13g Fiber 0g Protein 9g	1 cup skim milk

DAY 7
1,300 Calories

Meal/Snack Nutrition Data	Menu
Breakfast Calories 371 Fat 13g Saturated Fat 3g Sodium 570mg Carbohydrate 45g Fiber 4g Protein 20g	Breakfast Burrito: 1 egg scrambled in 1 tsp canola oil with chopped bell pepper and yellow onion, topped with 1 Tbsp salsa and 1 Tbsp shredded reduced-fat sharp cheddar cheese; wrapped in a 6-inch flour tortilla 1 cup nonfat milk ½ medium apple
Morning Snack Calories Fat Saturated Fat Sodium Carbohydrate Fiber Protein	None
Lunch Calories 375 Fat 13g Saturated Fat 1g Sodium 558mg Carbohydrate 51g Fiber 7g Protein 15g	1 cup Crunchy Fruit and Cabbage Slaw 1 small whole-wheat flatbread, such as Flatout Mini Harvest Wheat, filled with 2 Tbsp hummus, grated carrot, chopped cucumber, and red onion 1 cup nonfat milk
Afternoon Snack Calories 100 Fat 3g Saturated Fat 0g Sodium 30mg Carbohydrate 9g Fiber 4g Protein 8g	½ cup edamame beans in the pod (lightly salted, if desired)
Dinner Calories 495 Fat 19g Saturated Fat 3g Sodium 766mg Carbohydrate 51g Fiber 8g Protein 31g	1⅓ cups Chicken Stir-Fry with Broccoli and Tomatoes ⅔ cup brown rice with 2 tsp reduced-calorie vegetable oil spread 1½ cups spring lettuce mix with 2 Tbsp light Italian dressing 1 medium plum

DAY 7
1,800 Calories

Meal/Snack Nutrition Data	Menu
Breakfast Calories 457 Fat 17g Saturated Fat 5g Sodium 630mg Carbohydrate 52g Fiber 5g Protein 25g	Breakfast Burrito: 2 eggs scrambled in 1 tsp canola oil with chopped bell pepper and yellow onion, topped with 1 Tbsp salsa and 1 Tbsp shredded reduced-fat sharp cheddar cheese; wrapped in a 6-inch flour tortilla 1 cup nonfat milk 1 small apple
Morning Snack Calories 219 Fat 13g Saturated Fat 2g Sodium 0mg Carbohydrate 23g Fiber 5g Protein 7g	49 pistachios in the shell 1 peach
Lunch Calories 400 Fat 15g Saturated Fat 1g Sodium 638mg Carbohydrate 54g Fiber 8g Protein 16g	1 cup Crunchy Fruit and Cabbage Slaw 1 small whole-wheat flatbread, such as Flatout Mini Harvest Wheat, filled with 3 Tbsp hummus, grated carrot, chopped cucumber, and red onion 1 cup nonfat milk
Afternoon Snack Calories 200 Fat 6g Saturated Fat 0g Sodium 60mg Carbohydrate 18g Fiber 8g Protein 16g	1 cup edamame beans in the pod (lightly salted if desired)
Dinner Calories 569 Fat 19g Saturated Fat 3g Sodium 590mg Carbohydrate 68g Fiber 10g Protein 33g	1⅓ cups Chicken Stir-Fry with Broccoli and Tomatoes 1 cup brown rice with 2 tsp reduced-calorie vegetable oil spread 1½ cups spring lettuce mix with 2 Tbsp light Italian dressing 1 medium plum

RECIPE APPENDIX

Breakfast

Breakfast Pizza

Mixed Berry Smoothie

Soup

Curry Roasted Cauliflower Soup

Rita's New England Clam Chowder

Side Dishes

Crunchy Fruit and Cabbage Slaw

Grilled Fresh Mission Figs

Lemon-Spiked Roasted Cauliflower

Lemony Asparagus Spear Salad

Veggie-Packed Potato Salad

Main Dishes

Asian Salmon

Bean and Barley Salad

Chicken Stir-Fry with Broccoli and Tomatoes

Chunky Greek-Style Salad with Tuna

Crispy Chicken Dijon

Fish en Papillote

Judy's Lightened Meatloaf

Salmon Fillets with Pineapple Salsa

Sautéed Scallops

Soft Turkey Tacos

Quinoa-Stuffed Peppers

Vegetarian Chili

Breakfast Pizza

1 whole-wheat English muffin
2 Tbsp low-sodium pasta sauce
½ ounce reduced-sodium ham, diced or torn into small pieces
2 Tbsp part-skim shredded mozzarella cheese
1 Roma tomato, diced
⅛ tsp dried oregano
Dash garlic powder

1. Preheat oven to 450°F. Place the English muffin on a baking sheet and bake for 5 minutes.
2. Layer the ingredients evenly over the two halves of the English muffin in the following order: pasta sauce, ham, cheese, tomato, oregano, and garlic powder.
3. Return to the oven for another 7–10 minutes until well melted and heated through.

Yield: 2 halves / Serves: 1 / Serving Size: 2 halves
Exchanges/Choices: 2 Starch, ½ Vegetable, 1 Lean Meat
Calories: 225 / Calories from Fat: 47
Total Fat: 5g / Saturated Fat: 2g / Trans Fat: 0g / Cholesterol: 14mg / Sodium: 469mg /
Total Carbohydrate: 34g / Dietary Fiber: 6g / Sugars: 11g / Protein: 13g

Mixed Berry Smoothie

1 cup plain nonfat Greek yogurt
1 cup frozen mixed berries or frozen mixed berries with cherries
1 Tbsp sucralose or sweetener of choice
2 Tbsp nonfat milk

1. Place all ingredients in a blender or a container for an immersion blender. Process until smooth. If you are not using frozen fruit, you will need to add several ice cubes to make the smoothie thick.

Yield: 1½ cups / Serves: 1 / Serving Size: 1½ cups
Exchanges/Choices: 1 Milk, 1 Fruit
Calories: 203 / Calories from Fat: 5
Total Fat: 1g / Saturated Fat: 0g / Trans Fat: 0g / Cholesterol: 0mg / Sodium: 101mg /
Total Carbohydrate: 30g / Dietary Fiber: 5g / Sugars: 21g / Protein: 22g

Curry Roasted Cauliflower Soup

Created by Wendy Jo Peterson, MS, RD, Owner of San Diego–based
  Edible Nutrition & Fuelin' Roadie

1 large cauliflower, stalk and florets cut into bite-sized pieces
1 tsp cumin
1 tsp coriander
2 tsp paprika
2 tsp curry powder
Zest of 1 lemon, wedges reserved
2 Tbsp olive oil
¼ cup red wine vinegar
32 ounces low sodium chicken broth

1. Preheat oven to 425°F.
2. In a large bowl, whisk together cumin, coriander, paprika, curry powder, lemon zest, olive oil, and red wine vinegar. Pour cauliflower into bowl and toss until coated. Pour mixture onto a heavy baking sheet and bake for 45 minutes.
3. Meanwhile, in a 4-quart stockpot, heat chicken broth over medium heat. Add the roasted cauliflower. Using an immersion blender (if using a food processor, process in batches to avoid spillage), blend until desired consistency is reached. Serve soup with lemon wedges on the side.

Yield: about 5 cups / Serves: 4 / Serving Size: about 1¼ cups
Exchanges/Choices: 2 Vegetable, 1½ Fat
Calories: 140 / Calories from Fat: 69
Total Fat: 8g / Saturated Fat: 1g / Trans Fat: 0g / Cholesterol: 0mg / Sodium: 136mg /
Total Carbohydrate: 13g / Dietary Fiber: 6g / Sugars: 4g / Protein: 7g

Rita's New England Clam Chowder

Created by Rita Grandgenett, MS, RD, of RD Associates of Michigan, Battle Creek, Michigan

2 6½-ounce cans minced clams, drained, juice reserved
1 cup chopped onion
1 Tbsp cooking oil
3 medium celery stalks, diced (about 1 cup)
2 cups chopped cauliflower
1 tsp reduced-sodium Worcestershire sauce
½ tsp dried thyme
1 tsp dried parsley
⅛ tsp pepper
1 bay leaf
3 cups 1% low-fat milk
2½ Tbsp whole-wheat flour

1. Pour the reserved clam juice into a measuring cup. Add enough water to measure 1 cup and put aside.
2. In a large saucepan, sauté the onion in the oil over medium-high heat for 5 minutes or until translucent. Add the clam juice, celery, cauliflower, Worcestershire sauce, thyme, parsley, pepper, and bay leaf. Bring to a boil. Reduce heat, cover, and simmer for 10 minutes or until vegetables are tender.
3. In a medium bowl, whisk the milk and flour until smooth. Add to the vegetable mixture, and increase the heat to medium. Cook until slightly thickened and bubbly, about 5–10 minutes. Stir occasionally to prevent scorching. Do not allow the soup to come to a full boil. Stir in the clams. Reduce the heat to medium-low and continue cooking for 1–2 minutes. Remove the bay leaf and serve.

Yield: 6 cups / Serves: 6 / Serving Size: 1 cup
Exchanges/Choices: ½ Fat Free Milk, 1 Vegetable, 1 Lean Meat, ½ Fat
Calories: 132 / Calories from Fat: 34
Total Fat: 4g / Saturated Fat: 1g / Trans Fat: 0g / Cholesterol: 19mg / Sodium: 494mg /
Total Carbohydrate: 15g / Dietary Fiber: 2g / Sugars: 8 / Protein: 11g

Crunchy Fruit and Cabbage Slaw

1-pound bag coleslaw mix (such as Dole)
1½ cups quartered grapes (about 8 ounces)
15-ounce can no-sugar-added mandarin oranges, drained and cut in half
1½ Tbsp canola oil
4 Tbsp apple cider vinegar
4 Tbsp packed brown sugar
¼ tsp salt
¼ tsp black pepper
⅔ cup chopped pecans

1. In a large bowl, combine the slaw, grapes, and oranges.
2. In a small bowl, whisk together the oil, vinegar, sugar, salt, and pepper.
3. Pour the dressing over the slaw and mix gently. Refrigerate several hours. Mix in the pecans before serving.

Yield: 8 cups / Serves: 8 / Serving Size: 1 cup
Exchanges/Choices: 2 Fat, ½ Fruit, ½ Other Carbohydrate, 1 Vegetable
Calories: 154 / Calories from Fat: 82
Total Fat: 9g / Saturated Fat: 1g / Trans Fat: 0g / Cholesterol: 0mg / Sodium: 118mg /
Total Carbohydrate: 18g / Dietary Fiber: 2g / Sugars: 14g / Protein: 2g

Grilled Fresh Mission Figs

From *The All-Natural Diabetes Cookbook*, by Jackie Newgent, RD

6 medium fresh Black Mission figs
1 tsp aged balsamic vinegar
1 tsp acacia or orange blossom honey
2 tsp thinly sliced fresh mint

1. Lightly coat a grill or grill pan with natural cooking spray.
2. Preheat grill or grill pan over medium-high heat.
3. Remove stems from the figs and slice in half vertically.
4. Brush the cut surface of the figs with vinegar.
5. Grill, cut side down, for about 3 minutes or until charred.
6. Drizzle with honey and top with mint.

Yield: 12 halves / Serves: 4 / Serving Size: 3 halves
Exchanges/Choices: ½ Fruit
Calories: 40 / Calories from Fat: 0
Total Fat: 0g / Saturated Fat: 0g / Trans Fat: 0g / Cholesterol: 0mg / Sodium: 0mg /
Total Carbohydrate: 10g / Dietary Fiber: 1g / Sugars: 8g / Protein: 0g

Lemon-Spiked Roasted Cauliflower

2 Tbsp olive oil
1½ Tbsp lemon juice
1 clove garlic, crushed or chopped
¼ tsp kosher salt
⅛ tsp black pepper or to taste
1 Tbsp chopped fresh dill, divided
1 medium head cauliflower, trimmed and cut into 1½-inch pieces, dried well

1. Preheat oven to 450°F. In a large bowl, whisk together olive oil, lemon juice, garlic, salt, pepper, and ½ Tbsp dill. Add the cauliflower to the bowl and toss.
2. In a large pan, place the cauliflower in a single layer with the cut side down. Be careful to leave excess vinaigrette in the bowl and to avoid crowding the pan. Place into the preheated oven. After 10 minutes, turn the cauliflower and continue cooking for another 6 minutes or until tender and brown. Once done, transfer to a serving dish and sprinkle with the remaining dill.

Yield: about 2½–3 cups / Serves: 4 / Serving Size: about ⅔ cup
Exchanges/Choices: 1½ Vegetable, 1½ Fat
Calories: 99 / Calories from Fat: 64
Total Fat: 7g / Saturated Fat: 1g / Trans Fat: 0g / Cholesterol: 0mg / Sodium: 164mg /
Total Carbohydrate: 8g / Dietary Fiber: 3g / Sugars: 3g / Protein: 3g

Lemony Asparagus Spear Salad

From *The 4-Ingredient Diabetes Cookbook*, by Nancy S. Hughes

1 lb asparagus spears, trimmed
1 Tbsp basil pesto sauce
2 Tbsp lemon juice
¼ tsp salt

1. Cover asparagus with water in a 12-inch skillet and bring to a boil, then cover tightly and cook 1 minute or until tender-crisp.
2. Immediately drain the asparagus in a colander and run under cold water to cool. Place the asparagus on paper towels to drain, then place on a serving platter. Top the asparagus with the pesto and roll the spears back and forth to coat completely.
3. Drizzle with lemon juice and sprinkle with salt. Flavors are at their peak if you serve this within 30 minutes. You can cook the asparagus ahead of time and refrigerate it, but wait until serving time to add the remaining ingredients.

Yield: about 20 spears / Serves: 4 / Serving Size: 5 spears
Exchanges/Choices: 1 Vegetable, ½ Fat
Calories: 40 / Calories from Fat: 19
Total Fat: 2g / Saturated Fat: 1g / Trans fat: 0g / Cholesterol: 1mg / Sodium: 180mg /
Total Carbohydrate: 4g / Dietary Fiber: 1g / Sugars: 1g / Protein: 3g

Veggie-Packed Potato Salad

1½ lb red-skinned potatoes, cut into large bite-sized pieces
4 ounces snow peas, trimmed and cut into bite-sized pieces (about 1¼ cups)
3 Tbsp olive oil
3 Tbsp seasoned rice vinegar
½ tsp kosher salt
⅛–¼ tsp black pepper
1 tsp Dijon mustard
4 scallions, chopped (about ½ cup)
1 cup chopped red or orange bell pepper
½ cup chopped parsley

1. Place the potatoes in a large saucepan and cover with water. Bring to a boil, then reduce heat so the water bubbles gently. Cook until potatoes are nearly at desired tenderness, about 10 minutes, but test them frequently to avoid over-cooking. Just before the potatoes are done, drop the snow peas in the pot and cook for 30–60 seconds, until they are slightly softer but still crunchy. Drain and rinse in cold water to stop the cooking process.
2. While the potatoes are cooking, whisk the oil, vinegar, salt, black pepper, and mustard together.
3. Once the potatoes and snow peas are well drained, put them in a large bowl with the scallions, bell pepper, and parsley. Pour the dressing over the potatoes and vegetables and mix gently. Chill well before serving.

Yield: about 7 cups / Serves: 6 / Serving Size: about 1⅛ cups
Exchanges/Choices: 1 Starch, 1 Vegetable, 1½ Fat
Calories: 167 / Calories from Fat: 63
Total Fat: 7g / Saturated Fat: 1g / Trans Fat: 0g / Cholesterol: 0mg / Sodium: 354mg /
Total Carbohydrate: 24g / Dietary Fiber: 3g / Sugars: 5g / Protein: 3g

Asian Salmon

2 tsp canola oil
1½–2 tsp jarred or freshly minced ginger
4 4-ounce salmon fillets
4 tsp sesame oil
2 Tbsp and 2 tsp (8 tsp) reduced-sodium soy sauce
4 scallions, chopped

1. Preheat oven to 350°F. Mix the canola oil and ginger together, and spread evenly over the salmon.
2. Bake 20 minutes or until cooked through. Generally allow 10 minutes per inch of thickness. Meanwhile mix the sesame oil and soy sauce together.
3. Before serving, mix the scallions into the sesame oil–soy sauce mixture, pour over the cooked salmon, and serve.

Yield: 4 salmon fillets / Serves: 4 / Serving Size: 1 salmon fillet with ¼ of the sesame-soy-scallion mixture
Exchanges/Choices: 3 Lean Meat, 2½ Fat
Calories: 309 / Calories from Fat: 198
Total Fat: 22g / Saturated Fat: 4g / Trans Fat: 0g / Cholesterol: 62mg / Sodium: 473mg / Total Carbohydrate: 2g / Dietary Fiber: 0g / Sugars: 0g / Protein: 24g

Bean and Barley Salad

2 cups cooked pearled barley (prepared without salt)
3 ounces baby spinach, torn (about 4–5 cups whole baby spinach leaves), remove tough stems if any
1 6-ounce jar marinated artichoke hearts, drained and chopped (about ¾ cup chopped)
1 cup cherry tomatoes, halved (about 5–6 ounces)
1 15-ounce can no salt added cannellini beans, rinsed and drained
3 Tbsp olive oil
3 Tbsp lemon juice
1 clove garlic, crushed or chopped
¼ tsp black pepper
2 ounces reduced-fat feta cheese, crumbled

1. In a large bowl, mix together the cooked barley, spinach, artichoke hearts, tomatoes, and beans.
2. In a small bowl, mix together the oil, lemon juice, garlic, and pepper.
3. Pour the dressing over the barley, beans, and vegetables and mix well. Chill several hours. Before serving, sprinkle with the feta cheese and mix gently.

Yield: 8 cups / Serves: 6 / Serving Size: about 1⅓ cups
Exchanges/Choices: 1 Vegetable, 1½ Starch, 1 Lean Meat, 1½ Fat
Calories: 230 / Calories from Fat: 87
Total Fat: 10g / Saturated Fat: 2g / Trans Fat: 0g / Cholesterol: 3mg / Sodium: 241mg /
Total Carbohydrate: 30g / Dietary Fiber: 7g / Sugars: 2g / Protein: 8g

Chicken Stir-Fry with Broccoli and Tomatoes

5 cups fresh broccoli florets (about 10 ounces)
5 tsp canola oil, divided
½ cup chopped scallions
2–3 Tbsp reduced-sodium chicken broth
2 cloves garlic, crushed or chopped
1 lb boneless, skinless chicken breast, cut into bite-sized pieces
¼ tsp salt
⅛ tsp black pepper
1 cup cherry tomatoes, cut in half
2 Tbsp reduced-sodium soy sauce

1. Bring a pot of water to a boil and plunge the broccoli for 1–2 minutes to blanch. Drain. Plunge into a bowl of very cold water and drain again.
2. Heat a large skillet over high heat. Add 2 tsp oil. Once the oil is heated, add the scallions and broccoli, stirring quickly to coat with oil. Continue cooking for 1–3 minutes until desired tenderness is reached. Deglaze the pan with 1 Tbsp chicken broth, if necessary. Turn the heat to medium, and remove the vegetables. Keep warm.
3. Add the remaining 3 tsp oil. Add the garlic; stir. Add the chicken. Increase the heat to high, and cook about 1 minute without disturbing. Sprinkle the chicken with salt and pepper, and stir. Cook 2–5 minutes or until chicken is golden and cooked through. While the chicken is cooking, add 2 Tbsp chicken broth, scraping the bottom of the pan to lift the tiny brown bits of chicken.
4. Return the vegetables to the pan. Add the tomatoes; stir. Turn the heat to medium, cover, and continue cooking until the tomatoes are soft and release their juices. Stir occasionally, scraping the bottom of the pan and gently pressing on the tomatoes with a spatula. Remove the chicken and vegetables to a serving dish and sprinkle with soy sauce.

Yield: 5½ cups / Serves: 4 / Serving Size: about 1⅓ cups
Exchanges/Choices: 3 Lean Meat, 1½ Vegetable, 1 Fat
Calories: 215 / Calories from Fat: 79
Total Fat: 9g / Saturated Fat: 1g / Trans Fat: 0g / Cholesterol: 63mg / Sodium: 438mg /
Total Carbohydrate: 8g / Dietary Fiber: 3g / Sugars: 2g / Protein: 26g

Chunky Greek-Style Salad with Tuna

From *One Pot Meals for People with Diabetes, 2nd Edition*, by Ruth Glick and
   Nancy Baggett

3 Tbsp olive oil
½ Tbsp red wine vinegar
½ tsp dried thyme leaves
½ tsp dried basil leaves
½ cup crumbled reduced-fat feta cheese
6 cups mixed salad greens
5 oil-cured pitted Greek olives, seeded and chopped
1 small cucumber, peeled and cubed
2 Tbsp sliced green onion
1 medium tomato, cubed
6-oz can water-packed albacore tuna, well drained
1 cup seasoned croutons

1. In a large bowl, combine oil, vinegar, thyme, and basil. Stir to mix well.
2. Stir in the cheese. Add the greens, olives, cucumber, onion, and tomato. Toss
   to coat with dressing.
3. Add the tuna and croutons; toss. Serve immediately.

Yield: about 7½ cups / Serves: 5 / Serving Size: 1½ cups
Exchange/Choices: 2 Vegetable, 1½ Lean Meat, 1 Fat
Calories: 191 / Calories from Fat: 99
Total Fat: 11g / Saturated Fat: 2g / Trans Fat: 0g / Cholesterol: 24mg / Sodium: 428mg
/ Total Carbohydrate: 10g / Dietary Fiber: 2g / Sugars: 2g / Protein: 13g

Crispy Chicken Dijon

From *Lickety-Split Diabetic Meals*, by Zonya Foco, RD, CHFI, CSP

2 (8 oz each) sweet potatoes or 4 baking potatoes (4 oz each)
10-oz package frozen green beans, broccoli, or pea pods
10-oz package frozen sliced carrots
½ cup dry bread crumbs, unseasoned
¼ cup Dijon mustard
1 Tbsp olive oil
4 (4 oz each) boneless, skinless chicken breasts
   or 16 oz extra-firm tofu, cut into 8½-inch slices

1. Scrub potatoes thoroughly and pierce three or four times with a fork. Wrap in a damp paper towel.
2. Place in microwave for 12 minutes on high. Test doneness by piercing with a fork.
3. Place steamer basket in a pan and add 1 inch of water. Place over medium-high heat. Add vegetables and cover. Boil for 8 minutes.
4. Take out two cereal bowls and place bread crumbs in one and mustard in the other.
5. Add oil to medium nonstick skillet and heat over medium heat.
6. Dip chicken in mustard, then roll in the crumbs.
7. Brown each side of the chicken in the skillet, 4–5 minutes, until cooked all the way through. If vegetable timer goes off before you're ready, remove from heat and partially remove lid.

Yield: 4 breasts, 2 sweet potatoes, and 4 cups vegetables / Serves: 4 / Serving Size: 1 chicken breast, ½ sweet potato, and 1 cup vegetables
Exchanges/Choices: 2 Starch, 1 Vegetable, 4 Lean Meat
Calories: 325 / Calories from Fat: 52
Total Fat: 6g / Saturated Fat: 1g / Trans Fat: 0g / Cholesterol: 92mg / Sodium: 573mg /
Total Carbohydrate: 28g / Dietary Fiber: 2g / Sugars: 4g / Protein: 33g

Fish en Papillote

4 fillets rockfish, snapper, or grouper (each about 5–6 ounces)
2 small zucchini, cut into pieces about 3" x ¾"
  (will overcook if you cut them too small)
1 medium carrot, cut into matchsticks or shaved with a vegetable peeler
1 Tbsp olive oil
1 clove garlic, crushed or chopped
½ tsp kosher salt
¼ tsp black pepper
2 Tbsp chopped fresh chives
2 Tbsp capers
1 lime, thinly sliced

1. Preheat oven to 400°F. Take four 24-inch pieces of parchment paper. Folding each in half crosswise, cut them into heart shapes so that the fold is the center of the heart. On one half of the parchment paper, place the fish on top of a mound of zucchini and carrot.
2. Mix the oil and garlic together and drizzle over the fish. Sprinkle with salt, pepper, chives, and capers. Layer the lime slices on top of the fish. Fold the parchment paper over the ingredients and seal by overlapping the edges. Place each packet on a baking sheet.
3. Bake until the parchment paper has puffed up and the fish is cooked through, about 15–20 minutes. Place one packet on each of four plates and serve.

Yield: 4 fillets / Serves: 4 / Serving Size: 1 fillet
Exchanges/Choices: 4 Lean Meat, 1 Vegetable, 1 Fat
Calories: 207 / Calories from Fat: 53
Total Fat: 6g / Saturated Fat: 1g / Trans Fat: 0g / Cholesterol: 85mg / Sodium: 509mg /
Total Carbohydrate: 6g / Dietary Fiber: 2g / Sugars: 2g / Protein: 32g

Judy's Lightened Meatloaf

Created by Judy Doherty, Food and Health Communications
(*http://foodandhealth.com*)

1 lb frozen stew vegetables (combination of carrots, celery, onions,
    and potatoes)
6-ounce can tomato paste
1 lb 95% lean ground beef
2 egg whites
½ tsp onion powder
½ tsp garlic powder
¼ tsp black pepper
¼ tsp dried oregano
½ tsp kosher salt
1 cup whole-wheat bread crumbs
2 Tbsp ketchup

1. Preheat the oven to 375°F. Place the frozen vegetables in ¼ cup water in the microwave and cook on high for 10 minutes or until very tender. Drain. Purée them with the tomato paste in a food processor until smooth.
2. Mix the beef, vegetable purée, egg whites, seasonings, and bread crumbs together in a large bowl. Place into a loaf pan that has been sprayed with non-stick cooking spray. Top with ketchup and bake for 1 hour.
3. Allow the meatloaf to sit for 10 minutes before cutting into eight slices. This is a very soft meatloaf, so you may need to use both a spatula and a knife or two spatulas to lift the slice intact.

Yield: 1 loaf / Serves: 8 / Serving Size: ⅛ loaf
Exchanges/Choices: ½ Starch, 2 Vegetable, 2 Lean Meat
Calories: 180 / Calories from Fat: 32
Total Fat: 4g / Saturated Fat: 1g / Trans Fat: 0g / Cholesterol: 35mg / Sodium: 501mg /
Total Carbohydrate: 19g / Dietary Fiber: 3g / Sugars: 6g / Protein: 16g

Salmon Fillets with Pineapple Salsa

From *15-Minute Diabetic Meals*, by Nancy S. Hughes

4 4-oz salmon fillets, rinsed and patted dry
½ tsp dried thyme leaves
15¼-ounce can pineapple tidbits, packed in juice, drained
½ cup finely chopped red bell pepper
¼ cup finely chopped red onion
1 tsp grated ginger
⅛ tsp dried red pepper flakes (optional)

1. Line a baking sheet with foil, coat with cooking spray, and place the salmon, skin side down, on baking sheet. Sprinkle fish with thyme and season lightly with salt and pepper, if desired. Broil 10 minutes or until fish flakes.
2. Meanwhile, in a small bowl, combine all remaining ingredients to prepare a salsa. Set aside.
3. Serve the salmon with the salsa alongside.

Yield: 4 fillets and 2 cups salsa / Serves: 4 / Serving Size: 3 oz cooked fillet and about ½ cup salsa
Exchange/Choices: 1 Fruit, 4 Lean Meat, ½ Fat
Calories: 225 / Calories from Fat: 90
Total Fat: 10g / Saturated Fat: 1.8g / Trans Fat: 0g / Cholesterol: 80mg / Sodium: 60mg / Total Carbohydrate: 15g / Dietary Fiber: 2g / Sugars: 12g / Protein: 26g

Sautéed Scallops

1 lb scallops
1 Tbsp and 1 tsp olive oil, divided
1 Tbsp lemon juice
1 clove garlic, crushed or chopped
¼ tsp kosher salt
¼ tsp black pepper
¼ tsp dried thyme leaves
1 Tbsp fresh chives

1. Toss the scallops briefly with 1 tsp olive oil, lemon juice, garlic, salt, pepper, and thyme. Do not marinate.
2. Heat the remaining 1 Tbsp olive oil in a large nonstick skillet over medium-high heat. Add the scallops and cook 2–3 minutes per side, longer if the scallops are very large.
3. Remove the scallops to a platter and sprinkle with chives.

Serves: 4 / Serving Size: ¼ recipe
Exchanges/Choices: 2 Lean Meat, 1 Fat
Calories: 121 / Calories from Fat: 45
Total Fat: 5g / Saturated Fat: 1g / Trans Fat: 0g / Cholesterol: 27mg / Sodium: 565mg /
Total Carbohydrate: 4g / Dietary Fiber: 0g / Sugars: 0g / Protein: 14g

Soft Turkey Tacos

1 lb 93% lean ground turkey
1 large yellow onion, chopped
1 large red bell pepper, chopped
⅛ tsp kosher salt
⅛ tsp black pepper
1 tsp chili powder
1 tsp garlic powder
1 tsp dried oregano
½ tsp cumin
15-ounce can kidney beans, no salt added, drained and rinsed
12 6-inch flour tortillas
2 medium tomatoes, chopped (about 1½ cups)
6 Tbsp fat-free sour cream
6 Tbsp shredded 2% reduced-fat sharp cheddar cheese

1. Place the meat in a large, preheated nonstick skillet over medium-high heat. Break up the meat. Add the onion and bell pepper. Once the meat is browned, add the seasonings. Lower the heat to medium and cook until the vegetables are softened, about 8 minutes, stirring occasionally to prevent sticking. If necessary, deglaze the pan with 1–2 Tbsp water.
2. Add the beans and stir. Cook 1–2 minutes or until the beans are heated through.
3. Serve each plate with 2 tortillas; 1 cup meat, bean, and vegetable mixture; ¼ cup chopped tomato; 1 Tbsp sour cream; and 1 Tbsp cheese.

Yield: 6 cups of meat, bean, and vegetable mixture / Serves: 6 / Serving Size: 1 cup filling mixture, 2 tortillas, ¼ cup chopped tomato, 1 Tbsp cheese, and 1 Tbsp sour cream
Exchanges/Choices: 3 Starch, 1 Vegetable, 3 Lean Meat
Calories: 422 / Calories from Fat: 100
Total Fat: 11g / Saturated Fat: 3g / Trans Fat: 0g / Cholesterol: 50mg / Sodium: 485mg / Total Carbohydrate: 54g / Dietary Fiber: 9g / Sugars: 5g / Protein: 28g

Quinoa-Stuffed Peppers

4 bell peppers, use a variety of colors
1 Tbsp canola oil
1 cup chopped yellow onion
6 baby bella mushrooms or other medium-sized mushrooms, sliced
10-ounce package cooked frozen spinach, thawed and squeezed of
   excess water
2 cups cooked red quinoa, or other quinoa if you cannot find red
1 cup garbanzo beans
1 cup low-sodium pasta sauce, tomato basil, or other favorite variety, divided
¼ tsp black pepper
4 Tbsp shredded Parmesan cheese

1. Preheat oven to 400 F. Cut the peppers in half lengthwise and discard the
   seeds and membranes. Place peppers cut side down in a single layer in a large
   microwave-safe casserole dish or plate. Cover with a lid or wax paper. Microwave on high for 5 minutes to soften the peppers. Remove the peppers and
   dry the casserole dish and return the peppers to it or move the peppers to a
   fresh oven-safe pan.
2. Meanwhile, heat the oil in a skillet over medium-high heat and sauté the
   onions for 5 minutes. Then add the mushrooms and sauté until the vegetables
   are soft. Lower the heat if necessary to prevent scorching. Remove the pan
   from the heat and add the spinach. Mix. Then add the cooked quinoa, garbanzo beans, ½ cup pasta sauce, and black pepper.
3. Fill each half pepper with ⅛ of the quinoa mixture and top with the remaining pasta sauce.
4. Cover. Bake for 20 minutes. Remove the cover and sprinkle evenly with the
   Parmesan cheese. Broil 2–3 minutes or until the cheese is melted.

Yield: 8 stuffed pepper halves / Serves: 4 / Serving Size: 2 halves
Exchanges/Choices: 2 Starch, 1 Lean Meat, 3 Vegetable, 1 Fat
Calories: 331 / Calories from Fat: 78
Total Fat: 9g / Saturated Fat: 2g / Trans Fat: 0g / Cholesterol: 6mg / Sodium: 193mg /
Total Carbohydrate: 50g / Dietary Fiber: 11g / Sugars: 12g / Protein: 15g

Vegetarian Chili

1 Tbsp canola oil
1 large yellow onion, chopped
2 large carrots, chopped
1 large green bell pepper, chopped
2 cloves garlic, crushed or chopped
4.5-ounce can diced green chili peppers
14.5-ounce can diced tomatoes, no salt added, undrained
15-ounce can black beans, no salt added, drained and rinsed
15-ounce can kidney beans, no salt added, drained and rinsed
¼ tsp salt
½–1 tsp chili powder
½ tsp cumin
½ tsp dried oregano
2½ cups low-sodium vegetable broth
6 Tbsp fat-free sour cream
6 scallions, chopped
Cilantro, chopped for garnish

1. Heat the oil in a large pot over medium-high heat. Cook the onions, carrots, bell pepper, and garlic until soft, about 5 minutes. Stir to prevent sticking. Add the chili peppers, tomatoes, beans, and seasonings. Stir. Add the broth and stir some more. Reduce the heat, cover, and simmer 30 minutes.
2. Pour into serving bowls. Top with sour cream, scallions, and cilantro.

Yield: about 6.5 cups / Serves: 6 / Serving Size: about 1 cup
Exchanges/Choices: 1½ Starch, 3 Vegetable, 1 Lean Meat, ½ Fat
Calories: 206 / Calories from Fat: 25
Total Fat: 3g / Saturated Fat: 0g / Trans Fat: 0g / Cholesterol: 1mg / Sodium: 304mg /
Total Carbohydrate: 36g / Dietary Fiber: 13g / Sugars: 9g / Protein: 11g

References

American College of Sports Medicine, American Diabetes Association: Exercise and type 2 diabetes (Position Statement). *Med Sci Sports Exerc* 42:2282–2303, 2010

American Heart Association: Trans fats. Available from http://www.heart.org/HEARTORG/GettingHealthy/FatsAndOils/Fats101/Saturated-Fats_UCM_301120_Article.jsp. Accessed 13 Dec 2011

Arnold L, Mann JI, Ball MJ: Metabolic effects of alterations in meal frequency in type 2 diabetes. *Diabetes Care* 20:1651–1654, 1997

Behall KM, Scholfield DJ, Hallfrisch J: Comparison of hormone and glucose responses of overweight women to barley and oats. J Am Coll Nutr 24:182–188, 2005

Blatt AD, Roe LS, Rolls BJ: Hidden vegetables: an effective strategy to reduce energy intake and increase vegetable intake in adults. *Am J Clin Nutr* 93:756–763, 2011

Center for Nutrition Policy and Promotion (USDA): *Dietary Guidelines for Americans, 2010.* Available from http://www.cnpp.usda.gov/DGAs2010-PolicyDocument.htm. Accessed 13 Dec 2011

Colberg S, Zarabi I., et al.: Postprandial walking is better for lowering the glycemic effect of dinner than pre-dinner exercise in type 2 diabetic individuals. *J Am Med Dir Assoc* 10:394–397, 2009

Farshchi HR, et al.: Deleterious effects of omitting breakfast on insulin sensitivity and fasting lipid profiles in healthy lean women. *Am J Clin Nutr* 81:388–396, 2005

Flechtner-Mors M, Ditschuneit HH, et al.: Metabolic and weight loss effects of long-term dietary intervention in obese patients: four-year results. *Obes Res* 8:399–402, 2000

Gorin AA, Phelan S, Wing RR, Hill JO: Promoting long-term weight control: does dieting consistency matter? *Int J Obes Relat Metab Disord* 28:278–281, 2004

Hollis JF, Gullion CM, et al.: Weight loss during the intensive intervention phase of the Weight-Loss Maintenance Trial. *Am J Prev Med* 35:118–126, 2008

Institute of Medicine of the National Academies: Dietary reference intakes. Available from http://www.iom.edu/Global/News%20Announcements/~/media/C5CD2DD7840544979A549EC47E56A02B.ashx. Accessed 13 Dec 2011

International Food Information Council Foundation: IFIC review: sodium in food and health. Available from http://www.foodinsight.org/Resources/Detail.aspx?topic=IFIC_Review_Sodium_in_Food_and_Health. Accessed 13 Dec 2011

Kemps E, Tiggemann M: A cognitive experimental approach to understanding and reducing food cravings. *Curr Dir Psychol Sci* 19:86–90, 2010

Kerver JM, et al.: Meal and snack patterns are associated with dietary intake of energy and nutrients in US adults. *J Am Diet Assoc* 106:46–53, 2006

Leiden University: Sleep deprivation directly affects blood sugar levels (press release). Available from http://www.news.leiden.edu/news/lack-of-sleep-affects-blood-sugar-level.html. Accessed 13 December 2011

Leidy HJ, Tang M, et al.: The effects of consuming frequent, higher protein meals on appetite and satiety during weight loss in overweight/obese men. *Obesity* 19:818–824, 2011

Logue EE, Jarjoura DG, Sutton KS, Smucker WD, Baughman KR, Capers CF: Longitudinal relationship between elapsed time in the action stages of change and weight loss. *Obes Res* 12:1499–1508, 2004

McCrory MA, Howarth NC, et al.: Eating frequency and energy regulation in free-living adults consuming self-selected diets. *J Nutr* 141:148S–153S, 2011

National Weight Control Registry: NWCR facts. Available from http://nwcr.ws/Research/default.htm. Accessed 13 Dec 2011

Nedeltcheva AV, Kilkus JM, Imperial J, Kasza K, Schoeller DA, Penev PD: Sleep curtailment is accompanied by increased intake of calories from snacks. *Am J Clin Nutr* 89:123–133, 2009

Phelan S, Wyatt H, Hill JO, Wing RR: Are the eating and exercise habits of successful weight losers changing? *Obes Res* 14:710–716, 2006

Riccardi G, Giacco R, Rivellese AA: Dietary fat, insulin sensitivity and the metabolic syndrome. *Clin Nutr* 23:447–456, 2004

Rolls BJ, Roe LS, Meengs JS: Salad and satiety: energy density and portion size of a first-course salad affect energy intake at lunch. *J Am Diet Assoc* 104:1570–1576, 2004

Sabanayagam C, Shankar A: Sleep duration and cardiovascular disease: results from the National Health Interview Survey. *Sleep* 33:1037–1042, 2010

Science Daily: Chewing gum reduces snack cravings and decreases consumption of sweet snacks. Available from http://www.sciencedaily.com/releases/2009/04/090419133824.htm. Accessed 13 Dec 2011

Shick SM, Wing RR, Klem ML, McGuire MT, Hill JO, Seagle HM: Persons successful at long-term weight loss and maintenance continue to consume a low calorie, low fat diet. *J Am Diet Assoc* 98:408-413, 1998

University of North Carolina Chapel Hill: UNC study helps clarify link between high-fat diet and type 2 diabetes (press release). Available from http://www.med.unc.edu/www/news/2011/april/unc-study-helps-clarify-link-between-high-fat-diet-and-type-2-diabetes. Accessed 13 Dec 2011

Wansink B: *Mindless Eating: Why We Eat More Than We Think.* New York, Bantam Books, 2006

Wansink B, van Ittersum K, Painter JE: Ice cream illusions: bowl size, spoon size, and self-served portion sizes. *Am J Prev Med* 31:240–243, 2006

Weight-control Information Network: Binge eating disorder. Available from http://www.win.niddk.nih.gov/publications/binge.htm#howdoes. Accessed 13 Dec 2011

Whole Grains Council: What are the health benefits? Available from http://www.wholegrainscouncil.org/whole-grains-101/what-are-the-health-benefits. Accessed 13 Dec 2011

Wing RR, Phelan S: Long-term weight loss maintenance. *Am J Clin Nutr* 82:222S–225S, 2005

Wursch P, Pi-Sunyer FX: The role of viscous soluble fiber in the metabolic control of diabetes: a review with special emphasis on cereals rich in beta-glucan. *Diabetes Care* 20:1774–1780, 1997

Wyatt HR, Grunwald GK, Mosca CL, Klem ML, Wing RR, Hill JO: Long-term weight loss and breakfast in subjects in the National Weight Control Registry. *Obes Res* 10:78–82, 2002

Index

blood pressure, 139–140
Borg Rate of Perceived Exertion (RPE) Scale, 31, 102
breakfast, 27–29
breakfast pizza, 199
breathing exercise, 125
brown rice, 144

c

calories, 9–11, 55
carbohydrates
  counting, 13–14, 43–45
  limited carbohydrate snacks, 94–95
  monitoring, 10–11
  snacks, 60–61
cardiovascular disease, 90, 139–140
chicken Dijon (crispy), 212
chicken stir-fry with broccoli and tomatoes, 210
chili, 219
cholesterol, 139–140
ChooseMyPlate.gov, 9–10
chunky Greek-style salad with tuna, 211
community supported agriculture, 150
cooking
  benefits of, 55
  healthy strategies, 55–56
  techniques, resources, 57
  tips, 10
  tools, 57
cravings, 95–96
crispy chicken Dijon, 212
crunchy fruit and cabbage slaw, 203
curry roasted cauliflower soup, 201

d

DASH diet, 173
Diabetes Etiquette card, 119
diabetes support groups, 119

Dietary Guidelines for Americans, 13–14, 129
diet examination, 115–117
dietitians, 117
Distraction Kits, 96–97

e

eating. *see also* foods; meal planning
  binge, 109
  diet examination, 115–117
  healthful, 20–22
  mindful, 101
  triggers, 61, 63–64
edamame beans, 124
exercise
  benefits of, 14, 51
  breathing, 125
  cardiovascular, 30
  excuses, 51–52
  guidelines, 14, 30
  gyms, 103
  hypoglycemia, avoiding, 31–32
  negative self-talk, 52–54
  pedometers, 15–16, 133–134
  peripheral neuropathy (nerve disease), 16–17
  personal trainers, 102–103
  program components, 15
  proliferative retinopathy (eye disease), 16
  rating, 31, 77–78, 102, 133
  strength training, 46–47
  tips, 17, 52
eye disease (proliferative retinopathy), 16

f

fast food, take out, 69–70, 113
fat
  calorie relationship, 10
  monitoring, 10–11

Other Titles from the American Diabetes Association

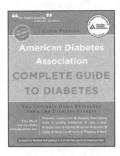

American Diabetes Association Complete Guide to Diabetes, 5th Edition
by American Diabetes Association
Have all of the tips and information on diabetes that you need close at hand. Complete with diagrams and easy-to-understand illustrations, sample medical forms, and an extensive list of resources, this guide breaks down how to live well with diabetes. The world's largest collection of diabetes self-care tips, techniques, and solutions to diabetes-related problems is back in its fifth edition, and it's bigger and better than ever before.
Order no. 4809-05; Price $22.95

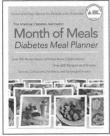

American Diabetes Association Month of Meals Diabetes Meal Planner
by American Diabetes Association
The bestselling Month of Meals™ series is all here—newly updated and collected into one complete, authoritative volume! Forget about the hassle of planning meals and spending hours making menus fit your diabetes management. With this invaluable guide, you'll have millions of daily menu combinations at your fingertips. Simply pick a menu for each meal, prepare your recipes, and enjoy a full day of delicious meals tailored specifically to you. It's as easy as that!
Order no. 4679-01; Price $22.95

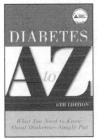

Diabetes A to Z, 6th Edition
by the American Diabetes Association
Diabetes jargon have you confused and perplexed? *Diabetes A to Z* is just what the doctor ordered. Get simple, informative answers to your questions. Medications, treatments, guidelines—they're all in here plus much more. Discover 50 vital categories that encompass everything from alcohol to vitamins to weight loss. Causes, treatments, definitions, and prevention tips all rolled into one.
Order no. 4801-06; Price $16.95

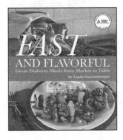

Fast and Flavorful
by Linda Gassenheimer
Do you love great, healthy meals bursting with flavor— but hate spending hours in the kitchen? Then you'll love *Fast and Flavorful*, a cookbook specially designed to get you out of the kitchen in record time. With handy shopping lists, helpful hints, and countdowns for preparing more than 120 incredible meals, you'll be dishing up healthy, diabetes-friendly dinners in minutes.
Order no. 4681-01; Price $18.95

To order these and other great American Diabetes Association titles, call **1-800-232-6733** or visit **http://shopdiabetes.org**. American Diabetes Association titles are also available in bookstores nationwide.

proliferative retinopathy (eye disease), 16